The Ultimate Congestive Heart Failure Cookbook

Nourishing Recipes to Revitalize Your Wellbeing, Step by step Guide to Nutritious Cooking for Congestive Heart Failure

Anita Hulsey

Table Of Contents

CHAPTER ONE

CHAPTER TWO

CHAPTER THREE

INTRODUCTION

Simon never thought he'd be writing a cookbook, let alone one focused on congestive heart failure. But after his own diagnosis a few years ago, he quickly realized the importance of a heart-healthy diet. Simon spent countless hours researching recipes, consulting with nutritionists, and tirelessly testing dishes in his kitchen. The result is this collection of Simon's favorite meals - all designed to nourish your heart and soul.

Congestive heart failure can feel overwhelming, but Simon is here to show you that delicious, nutritious meals are not only possible, but can actually be enjoyable. Within these pages, you'll find Simon's tips for managing symptoms, insight into the science behind a heart-healthy diet, and of course, mouthwatering recipes the whole family will love.

Simon knows firsthand that making dietary changes isn't easy. But with his warm, encouraging guidance, you'll be whipping up flavorful, doctor-approved dishes in no time. Get ready to rejuvenate your heart and taste buds with The Ultimate Congestive Heart Failure Cookbook.

CHAPTER ONE

Breakfast Recipes

Avocado Toast with Poached Eggs

Recipe 1:

Classic Avocado Toast with Poached Eggs

Ingredients:
- 2 slices whole grain bread, toasted
- 1 ripe avocado, mashed
- 2 large eggs, poached
- 1 tablespoon olive oil
- 1 tablespoon fresh lemon juice
- 1/4 teaspoon salt
- 1/8 teaspoon ground black pepper
- 2 tablespoons crumbled feta cheese (optional)

Nutritional Information (per serving):
- Calories: 325
- Total Fat: 19g
- Saturated Fat: 4g
- Carbohydrates: 29g
- Fiber: 9g
- Protein: 13g

Cooking Time: 15 minutes
Serving Size: 1 open-faced toast

Instructions:
1. Toast the whole grain bread.
2. In a small bowl, mash the avocado with the olive oil, lemon juice, salt, and pepper.
3. Spread the mashed avocado mixture evenly over the toasted bread slices.
4. Poach the eggs according to your preferred method.
5. Top each slice of avocado toast with a poached egg.
6. Optionally, sprinkle the crumbled feta cheese over the top.

7. Serve immediately.

Recipe 2:

Smashed Avocado Toast with Poached Eggs and Tomatoes

Ingredients:
- 2 slices whole grain bread, toasted
- 1 ripe avocado, mashed
- 2 large eggs, poached
- 1/2 cup cherry tomatoes, halved
- 1 tablespoon olive oil
- 1 tablespoon balsamic glaze
- 1/4 teaspoon salt
- 1/8 teaspoon ground black pepper

Nutritional Information (per serving):
- Calories: 350
- Total Fat: 21g
- Saturated Fat: 3g
- Carbohydrates: 31g
- Fiber: 9g
- Protein: 14g

Cooking Time: 15 minutes
Serving Size: 1 open-faced toast

Instructions:
1. Toast the whole grain bread.
2. In a small bowl, mash the avocado with the olive oil, salt, and pepper.
3. Spread the mashed avocado mixture evenly over the toasted bread slices.
4. Poach the eggs according to your preferred method.
5. Top each slice of avocado toast with a poached egg and the halved cherry tomatoes.
6. Drizzle the balsamic glaze over the top.
7. Serve immediately.

Recipe 3:

Spicy Avocado Toast with Poached Eggs and Microgreens

Ingredients:
- 2 slices whole grain bread, toasted

- 1 ripe avocado, mashed
- 2 large eggs, poached
- 1 tablespoon chipotle chili powder
- 1 tablespoon fresh lime juice
- 1/4 teaspoon salt
- 1/8 teaspoon ground black pepper
- 2 tablespoons microgreens or sprouts

Nutritional Information (per serving):
- Calories: 330
- Total Fat: 18g
- Saturated Fat: 3g
- Carbohydrates: 30g
- Fiber: 10g
- Protein: 14g

Cooking Time: 15 minutes
Serving Size: 1 open-faced toast

Instructions:
1. Toast the whole grain bread.
2. In a small bowl, mash the avocado with the chipotle chili powder, lime juice, salt, and pepper.

3. Spread the spicy avocado mixture evenly over the toasted bread slices.
4. Poach the eggs according to your preferred method.
5. Top each slice of avocado toast with a poached egg and the microgreens or sprouts.
6. Serve immediately.

Recipe 4:

Avocado Toast with Poached Eggs and Everything Bagel Seasoning

Ingredients:
- 2 slices whole grain bread, toasted
- 1 ripe avocado, mashed
- 2 large eggs, poached
- 2 tablespoons everything bagel seasoning
- 1 tablespoon olive oil
- 1 tablespoon fresh lemon juice
- 1/4 teaspoon salt
- 1/8 teaspoon ground black pepper

Nutritional Information (per serving):
- Calories: 340
- Total Fat: 20g
- Saturated Fat: 3g
- Carbohydrates: 31g
- Fiber: 9g
- Protein: 14g

Cooking Time: 15 minutes
Serving Size: 1 open-faced toast

Instructions:
1. Toast the whole grain bread.
2. In a small bowl, mash the avocado with the olive oil, lemon juice, salt, and pepper.
3. Spread the mashed avocado mixture evenly over the toasted bread slices.
4. Poach the eggs according to your preferred method.
5. Top each slice of avocado toast with a poached egg and a generous sprinkle of everything bagel seasoning.
6. Serve immediately.

Overnight Oats with Berries and Nuts

Recipe 1:

Blueberry Overnight Oats

Ingredients:
- 1 cup old-fashioned rolled oats
- 1 cup unsweetened almond milk
- 1/2 cup fresh or frozen blueberries
- 2 tablespoons chia seeds
- 1 tablespoon maple syrup
- 1/4 teaspoon ground cinnamon
- 2 tablespoons chopped walnuts

Nutritional Information (per serving):
- Calories: 310
- Total Fat: 12g
- Saturated Fat: 1g
- Carbohydrates: 44g
- Fiber: 9g
- Protein: 9g

Cooking Time: 5 minutes active, 8 hours refrigeration
Serving Size: 1 bowl

Instructions:
1. In a medium-sized bowl, combine the rolled oats, almond milk, blueberries, chia seeds, maple syrup, and cinnamon.
2. Stir well to combine, cover, and refrigerate for at least 8 hours, or overnight.
3. Top with the chopped walnuts before serving.

Recipe 2:

Strawberry Almond Overnight Oats

Ingredients:
- 1 cup old-fashioned rolled oats
- 1 cup unsweetened almond milk
- 1/2 cup fresh or frozen strawberries, chopped
- 2 tablespoons almond slivers
- 1 tablespoon honey

- 1/4 teaspoon vanilla extract

Nutritional Information (per serving):
- Calories: 295
- Total Fat: 10g
- Saturated Fat: 1g
- Carbohydrates: 45g
- Fiber: 7g
- Protein: 8g

Cooking Time: 5 minutes active, 8 hours refrigeration
Serving Size: 1 bowl

Instructions:
1. In a medium-sized bowl, combine the rolled oats, almond milk, chopped strawberries, almond slivers, honey, and vanilla extract.
2. Stir well to combine, cover, and refrigerate for at least 8 hours, or overnight.
3. Enjoy your Strawberry Almond Overnight Oats.

Recipe 3:

Mixed Berry Overnight Oats

Ingredients:
- 1 cup old-fashioned rolled oats
- 1 cup unsweetened almond milk
- 1/4 cup fresh or frozen mixed berries (such as blueberries, raspberries, and blackberries)
- 1 tablespoon chia seeds
- 1 tablespoon honey
- 1/4 teaspoon ground cardamom

Nutritional Information (per serving):
- Calories: 320
- Total Fat: 9g
- Saturated Fat: 1g
- Carbohydrates: 51g
- Fiber: 10g
- Protein: 9g

Cooking Time: 5 minutes active, 8 hours refrigeration
Serving Size: 1 bowl

Instructions:
1. In a medium-sized bowl, combine the rolled oats, almond milk, mixed berries, chia seeds, honey, and ground cardamom.
2. Stir well to combine, cover, and refrigerate for at least 8 hours, or overnight.
3. Enjoy your Mixed Berry Overnight Oats.

Recipe 4:

Peanut Butter and Banana Overnight Oats

Ingredients:
- 1 cup old-fashioned rolled oats
- 1 cup unsweetened almond milk
- 2 tablespoons creamy peanut butter
- 1 medium ripe banana, mashed
- 1 tablespoon maple syrup
- 1/4 teaspoon ground cinnamon
- 2 tablespoons chopped roasted peanuts

Nutritional Information (per serving):
- Calories: 385
- Total Fat: 16g
- Saturated Fat: 2g
- Carbohydrates: 52g
- Fiber: 8g
- Protein: 12g

Cooking Time: 5 minutes active, 8 hours refrigeration
Serving Size: 1 bowl

Instructions:
1. In a medium-sized bowl, combine the rolled oats, almond milk, peanut butter, mashed banana, maple syrup, and ground cinnamon.
2. Stir well to combine, cover, and refrigerate for at least 8 hours, or overnight.
3. Top with the chopped roasted peanuts before serving.

Spinach and Feta Frittata

Recipe 1:

Classic Spinach and Feta Frittata

Ingredients:
- 8 large eggs
- 1/4 cup unsweetened almond milk
- 1/2 teaspoon salt
- 1/4 teaspoon ground black pepper
- 1 tablespoon olive oil
- 2 cups fresh spinach, chopped
- 1/2 cup crumbled feta cheese

Nutritional Information (per serving):
- Calories: 190
- Total Fat: 13g
- Saturated Fat: 5g
- Carbohydrates: 4g
- Fiber: 1g
- Protein: 16g

Cooking Time: 25 minutes
Serving Size: 1/4 of the frittata

Instructions:
1. Preheat the oven to 375°F (190°C).
2. In a medium bowl, whisk together the eggs, almond milk, salt, and pepper.
3. Heat the olive oil in a 9-inch oven-safe skillet over medium heat.
4. Add the chopped spinach and sauté until wilted, about 2-3 minutes.
5. Pour the egg mixture over the spinach and sprinkle the crumbled feta cheese on top.
6. Transfer the skillet to the oven and bake for 18-20 minutes, or until the frittata is set.
7. Remove the frittata from the oven and let it cool for a few minutes before slicing and serving.

Recipe 2:

Spinach and Feta Frittata Muffins

Ingredients:
- 8 large eggs

- 1/4 cup unsweetened almond milk
- 1/2 teaspoon salt
- 1/4 teaspoon ground black pepper
- 1 tablespoon olive oil
- 2 cups fresh spinach, chopped
- 1/2 cup crumbled feta cheese

Nutritional Information (per serving):
- Calories: 170
- Total Fat: 12g
- Saturated Fat: 4g
- Carbohydrates: 3g
- Fiber: 1g
- Protein: 14g

Cooking Time: 25 minutes
Serving Size: 1 frittata muffin

Instructions:
1. Preheat the oven to 375°F (190°C). Grease a 12-cup muffin tin.
2. In a medium bowl, whisk together the eggs, almond milk, salt, and pepper.
3. Heat the olive oil in a skillet over medium heat. Add the chopped spinach

and sauté until wilted, about 2-3 minutes.
4. Divide the sautéed spinach evenly among the prepared muffin cups.
5. Pour the egg mixture over the spinach, filling each cup about 3/4 full.
6. Sprinkle the crumbled feta cheese on top of each frittata muffin.
7. Bake for 18-20 minutes, or until the frittatas are set and lightly golden.
8. Remove the frittata muffins from the oven and let them cool for a few minutes before serving.

Recipe 3:

Spinach and Feta Crustless Frittata

Ingredients:
- 10 large eggs
- 1/4 cup unsweetened almond milk
- 1/2 teaspoon salt
- 1/4 teaspoon ground black pepper
- 1 tablespoon olive oil
- 3 cups fresh spinach, chopped

- 3/4 cup crumbled feta cheese

Nutritional Information (per serving):
- Calories: 210
- Total Fat: 15g
- Saturated Fat: 6g
- Carbohydrates: 4g
- Fiber: 1g
- Protein: 18g

Cooking Time: 30 minutes
Serving Size: 1/6 of the frittata

Instructions:
1. Preheat the oven to 375°F (190°C). Grease a 9-inch pie dish or oven-safe skillet.
2. In a medium bowl, whisk together the eggs, almond milk, salt, and pepper.
3. Heat the olive oil in a skillet over medium heat. Add the chopped spinach and sauté until wilted, about 2-3 minutes.
4. Spread the sautéed spinach evenly in the prepared pie dish or skillet.

5. Pour the egg mixture over the spinach and sprinkle the crumbled feta cheese on top.

6. Bake for 25-30 minutes, or until the frittata is set and lightly golden.

7. Remove the frittata from the oven and let it cool for a few minutes before slicing and serving.

Recipe 4:

Spinach and Feta Frittata with Roasted Red Peppers

Ingredients:
- 8 large eggs
- 1/4 cup unsweetened almond milk
- 1/2 teaspoon salt
- 1/4 teaspoon ground black pepper
- 1 tablespoon olive oil
- 2 cups fresh spinach, chopped
- 1/2 cup crumbled feta cheese
- 1/2 cup roasted red peppers, chopped

Nutritional Information (per serving):

- Calories: 205
- Total Fat: 14g
- Saturated Fat: 5g
- Carbohydrates: 5g
- Fiber: 1g
- Protein: 16g

Cooking Time: 25 minutes
Serving Size: 1/4 of the frittata

Instructions:
1. Preheat the oven to 375°F (190°C).
2. In a medium bowl, whisk together the eggs, almond milk, salt, and pepper.
3. Heat the olive oil in a 9-inch oven-safe skillet over medium heat.
4. Add the chopped spinach and sauté until wilted, about 2-3 minutes.
5. Pour the egg mixture over the spinach and sprinkle the crumbled feta cheese and chopped roasted red peppers on top.
6. Transfer the skillet to the oven and bake for 18-20 minutes, or until the frittata is set.

7. Remove the frittata from the oven and let it cool for a few minutes before slicing and serving.

Whole Wheat Pancakes with Cinnamon Apples

Recipe 1:

Classic Whole Wheat Pancakes with Cinnamon Apples

Ingredients:
- 1 cup whole wheat flour
- 1 tablespoon baking powder
- 1/2 teaspoon ground cinnamon
- 1/4 teaspoon salt
- 1 cup unsweetened almond milk
- 1 large egg
- 1 tablespoon maple syrup
- 1 tablespoon unsalted butter, melted
- 2 medium apples, peeled, cored, and diced
- 1 teaspoon ground cinnamon

- 1 tablespoon maple syrup

Nutritional Information (per serving):
- Calories: 300
- Total Fat: 9g
- Saturated Fat: 3g
- Carbohydrates: 48g
- Fiber: 6g
- Protein: 9g

Cooking Time: 25 minutes
Serving Size: 2 pancakes with 1/4 cup cinnamon apples

Instructions:
1. In a large bowl, whisk together the whole wheat flour, baking powder, 1/2 teaspoon cinnamon, and salt.
2. In a separate bowl, whisk together the almond milk, egg, 1 tablespoon maple syrup, and melted butter.
3. Add the wet ingredients to the dry ingredients and stir just until combined (do not overmix).

4. In a small saucepan, combine the diced apples, 1 teaspoon cinnamon, and 1 tablespoon maple syrup. Cook over medium heat, stirring occasionally, until the apples are softened, about 5-7 minutes.

5. Heat a large non-stick skillet or griddle over medium heat. Scoop 1/4 cup of batter per pancake and cook for 2-3 minutes per side, or until golden brown.

6. Serve the pancakes warm, topped with the cinnamon apples.

Recipe 2:

Fluffy Whole Wheat Pancakes with Cinnamon Apples

Ingredients:
- 1 1/4 cups whole wheat flour
- 2 teaspoons baking powder
- 1/2 teaspoon ground cinnamon
- 1/4 teaspoon salt
- 1 cup unsweetened almond milk

- 1 large egg
- 2 tablespoons maple syrup
- 1 tablespoon unsalted butter, melted
- 3 medium apples, peeled, cored, and diced
- 2 teaspoons ground cinnamon
- 2 tablespoons maple syrup

Nutritional Information (per serving):
- Calories: 320
- Total Fat: 10g
- Saturated Fat: 3g
- Carbohydrates: 53g
- Fiber: 7g
- Protein: 9g

Cooking Time: 30 minutes
Serving Size: 2 pancakes with 1/3 cup cinnamon apples

Instructions:
1. In a large bowl, whisk together the whole wheat flour, baking powder, 1/2 teaspoon cinnamon, and salt.

2. In a separate bowl, whisk together the almond milk, egg, 2 tablespoons maple syrup, and melted butter.

3. Add the wet ingredients to the dry ingredients and stir just until combined (do not overmix).

4. In a medium saucepan, combine the diced apples, 2 teaspoons cinnamon, and 2 tablespoons maple syrup. Cook over medium heat, stirring occasionally, until the apples are softened and syrupy, about 7-10 minutes.

5. Heat a large non-stick skillet or griddle over medium heat. Scoop 1/4 cup of batter per pancake and cook for 2-3 minutes per side, or until golden brown.

6. Serve the pancakes warm, topped with the cinnamon apples.

Recipe 3:

Whole Wheat Pancakes with Cinnamon Apples and Pecans

Ingredients:
- 1 1/2 cups whole wheat flour
- 1 1/2 teaspoons baking powder
- 1/2 teaspoon ground cinnamon
- 1/4 teaspoon salt
- 1 cup unsweetened almond milk
- 1 large egg
- 1 tablespoon maple syrup
- 1 tablespoon unsalted butter, melted
- 4 medium apples, peeled, cored, and diced
- 2 teaspoons ground cinnamon
- 1/4 cup chopped toasted pecans

Nutritional Information (per serving):
- Calories: 370
- Total Fat: 13g
- Saturated Fat: 4g
- Carbohydrates: 56g
- Fiber: 8g
- Protein: 10g

Cooking Time: 35 minutes

Serving Size: 2 pancakes with 1/2 cup cinnamon apples and 1 tablespoon pecans

Instructions:
1. In a large bowl, whisk together the whole wheat flour, baking powder, 1/2 teaspoon cinnamon, and salt.
2. In a separate bowl, whisk together the almond milk, egg, 1 tablespoon maple syrup, and melted butter.
3. Add the wet ingredients to the dry ingredients and stir just until combined (do not overmix).
4. In a medium saucepan, combine the diced apples, 2 teaspoons cinnamon, and 2 tablespoons water. Cook over medium heat, stirring occasionally, until the apples are softened and syrupy, about 10 minutes.
5. Heat a large non-stick skillet or griddle over medium heat. Scoop 1/4 cup of batter per pancake and cook for 2-3 minutes per side, or until golden brown.

6. Serve the pancakes warm, topped with the cinnamon apples and chopped toasted pecans.

Recipe 4:

Whole Wheat Pancakes with Cinnamon Apple Compote

Ingredients:
- 1 1/4 cups whole wheat flour
- 1 tablespoon baking powder
- 1 teaspoon ground cinnamon
- 1/4 teaspoon salt
- 1 cup unsweetened almond milk
- 1 large egg
- 1 tablespoon maple syrup
- 1 tablespoon unsalted butter, melted
- 5 medium apples, peeled, cored, and diced
- 1/4 cup maple syrup
- 1 teaspoon ground cinnamon

Nutritional Information (per serving):
- Calories: 340

- Total Fat: 9g
- Saturated Fat: 3g
- Carbohydrates: 59g
- Fiber: 7g
- Protein: 9g

Cooking Time: 40 minutes
Serving Size: 2 pancakes with 1/3 cup cinnamon apple compote

Instructions:
1. In a large bowl, whisk together the whole wheat flour, baking powder, 1 teaspoon cinnamon, and salt.
2. In a separate bowl, whisk together the almond milk, egg, 1 tablespoon maple syrup, and melted butter.
3. Add the wet ingredients to the dry ingredients and stir just until combined (do not overmix).
4. In a medium saucepan, combine the diced apples, 1/4 cup maple syrup, and 1 teaspoon cinnamon. Cook over medium heat, stirring occasionally, until the

apples are softened and the mixture has thickened, about 15-20 minutes.

5. Heat a large non-stick skillet or griddle over medium heat. Scoop 1/4 cup of batter per pancake and cook for 2-3 minutes per side, or until golden brown.

6. Serve the pancakes warm, topped with the cinnamon apple compote.

CHAPTER TWO

Lunch Recipes

Grilled Salmon Salad with Lemon Vinaigrette

Recipe 1:

Classic Grilled Salmon Salad with Lemon Vinaigrette

Ingredients:
- 4 (4-oz) salmon fillets
- 1 tablespoon olive oil
- 1/2 teaspoon salt
- 1/4 teaspoon ground black pepper
- 6 cups mixed greens
- 1 cup grape tomatoes, halved
- 1/2 cucumber, sliced
- 1/4 red onion, thinly sliced
- 2 tablespoons chopped fresh parsley

Lemon Vinaigrette:
- 2 tablespoons olive oil
- 2 tablespoons lemon juice
- 1 teaspoon Dijon mustard
- 1 teaspoon honey
- 1/4 teaspoon salt
- 1/8 teaspoon ground black pepper

Nutritional Information (per serving):
- Calories: 335
- Total Fat: 19g
- Saturated Fat: 3g
- Carbohydrates: 11g
- Fiber: 3g
- Protein: 31g

Cooking Time: 25 minutes
Serving Size: 1 salmon fillet with 1 1/2 cups salad and 2 tablespoons vinaigrette

Instructions:
1. Preheat grill or grill pan to medium-high heat.

2. Brush the salmon fillets with 1 tablespoon of olive oil and season with salt and pepper.
3. Grill the salmon for 3-4 minutes per side, or until it flakes easily with a fork.
4. In a large bowl, combine the mixed greens, grape tomatoes, cucumber, and red onion.
5. In a small bowl, whisk together the ingredients for the lemon vinaigrette.
6. Divide the salad among 4 plates and top each with a grilled salmon fillet.
7. Drizzle the lemon vinaigrette over the salad and salmon.
8. Sprinkle the chopped fresh parsley over the top.

Recipe 2:

Grilled Salmon Salad with Lemon Vinaigrette and Avocado

Ingredients:
- 4 (4-oz) salmon fillets
- 1 tablespoon olive oil

- 1/2 teaspoon salt
- 1/4 teaspoon ground black pepper
- 6 cups baby spinach
- 1 avocado, diced
- 1 cup sliced strawberries
- 1/4 cup crumbled feta cheese

Lemon Vinaigrette:
- 2 tablespoons olive oil
- 2 tablespoons lemon juice
- 1 teaspoon Dijon mustard
- 1 teaspoon honey
- 1/4 teaspoon salt
- 1/8 teaspoon ground black pepper

Nutritional Information (per serving):
- Calories: 375
- Total Fat: 24g
- Saturated Fat: 5g
- Carbohydrates: 14g
- Fiber: 5g
- Protein: 31g

Cooking Time: 25 minutes

Serving Size: 1 salmon fillet with 1 1/2 cups salad and 2 tablespoons vinaigrette

Instructions:
1. Preheat grill or grill pan to medium-high heat.
2. Brush the salmon fillets with 1 tablespoon of olive oil and season with salt and pepper.
3. Grill the salmon for 3-4 minutes per side, or until it flakes easily with a fork.
4. In a large bowl, combine the baby spinach, diced avocado, and sliced strawberries.
5. In a small bowl, whisk together the ingredients for the lemon vinaigrette.
6. Divide the salad among 4 plates and top each with a grilled salmon fillet.
7. Drizzle the lemon vinaigrette over the salad and salmon.
8. Sprinkle the crumbled feta cheese over the top.

Recipe 3:

Grilled Salmon Salad with Lemon Vinaigrette and Quinoa

Ingredients:
- 4 (4-oz) salmon fillets
- 1 tablespoon olive oil
- 1/2 teaspoon salt
- 1/4 teaspoon ground black pepper
- 4 cups mixed greens
- 1 cup cooked quinoa
- 1 cup diced cucumber
- 1/2 cup cherry tomatoes, halved
- 2 tablespoons chopped fresh basil

Lemon Vinaigrette:
- 3 tablespoons olive oil
- 2 tablespoons lemon juice
- 1 teaspoon Dijon mustard
- 1 teaspoon honey
- 1/4 teaspoon salt
- 1/8 teaspoon ground black pepper

Nutritional Information (per serving):
- Calories: 390
- Total Fat: 21g

- Saturated Fat: 3g
- Carbohydrates: 22g
- Fiber: 4g
- Protein: 32g

Cooking Time: 30 minutes
Serving Size: 1 salmon fillet with 1 cup salad and 2 tablespoons vinaigrette

Instructions:
1. Preheat grill or grill pan to medium-high heat.
2. Brush the salmon fillets with 1 tablespoon of olive oil and season with salt and pepper.
3. Grill the salmon for 3-4 minutes per side, or until it flakes easily with a fork.
4. In a large bowl, combine the mixed greens, cooked quinoa, diced cucumber, and cherry tomatoes.
5. In a small bowl, whisk together the ingredients for the lemon vinaigrette.
6. Divide the salad among 4 plates and top each with a grilled salmon fillet.

7. Drizzle the lemon vinaigrette over the salad and salmon.
8. Sprinkle the chopped fresh basil over the top.

Recipe 4:

Grilled Salmon Salad with Lemon Vinaigrette and Roasted Vegetables

Ingredients:
- 4 (4-oz) salmon fillets
- 1 tablespoon olive oil
- 1/2 teaspoon salt
- 1/4 teaspoon ground black pepper
- 1 cup roasted sweet potato cubes
- 1 cup roasted broccoli florets
- 4 cups baby arugula
- 1/4 cup toasted sliced almonds

Lemon Vinaigrette:
- 3 tablespoons olive oil
- 3 tablespoons lemon juice
- 1 teaspoon Dijon mustard
- 1 teaspoon honey

- 1/4 teaspoon salt
- 1/8 teaspoon ground black pepper

Nutritional Information (per serving):
- Calories: 425
- Total Fat: 26g
- Saturated Fat: 4g
- Carbohydrates: 18g
- Fiber: 5g
- Protein: 33g

Cooking Time: 35 minutes
Serving Size: 1 salmon fillet with 1 1/2 cups salad and 2 tablespoons vinaigrette

Instructions:
1. Preheat grill or grill pan to medium-high heat.
2. Brush the salmon fillets with 1 tablespoon of olive oil and season with salt and pepper.
3. Grill the salmon for 3-4 minutes per side, or until it flakes easily with a fork.

4. In a large bowl, combine the roasted sweet potato cubes, roasted broccoli florets, and baby arugula.
5. In a small bowl, whisk together the ingredients for the lemon vinaigrette.
6. Divide the salad among 4 plates and top each with a grilled salmon fillet.
7. Drizzle the lemon vinaigrette over the salad and salmon.
8. Sprinkle the toasted sliced almonds over the top.

Hearty Lentil and Vegetable Soup

Recipe 1:

Classic Hearty Lentil and Vegetable Soup

Ingredients:
- 1 tablespoon olive oil
- 1 large onion, diced
- 3 carrots, peeled and diced
- 3 celery stalks, diced

- 4 cloves garlic, minced
- 1 cup dried brown lentils, rinsed
- 6 cups vegetable broth
- 1 (14.5 oz) can diced tomatoes
- 2 cups chopped kale
- 1 teaspoon dried thyme
- 1 teaspoon dried oregano
- 1/2 teaspoon salt
- 1/4 teaspoon ground black pepper

Nutritional Information (per serving):
- Calories: 270
- Total Fat: 5g
- Saturated Fat: 1g
- Carbohydrates: 40g
- Fiber: 11g
- Protein: 16g

Cooking Time: 45 minutes
Serving Size: 1 1/2 cups

Instructions:
1. In a large pot or Dutch oven, heat the olive oil over medium heat.

2. Add the diced onion, carrots, and celery. Sauté for 5-7 minutes, until the vegetables are softened.
3. Stir in the minced garlic and cook for 1 minute, until fragrant.
4. Add the rinsed lentils, vegetable broth, diced tomatoes, chopped kale, thyme, oregano, salt, and pepper.
5. Bring the soup to a boil, then reduce the heat and simmer for 30-35 minutes, or until the lentils are tender.
6. Taste and adjust seasoning as needed.
7. Serve the soup hot, garnished with additional fresh herbs or a drizzle of olive oil, if desired.

Recipe 2:

Lentil and Vegetable Soup with Roasted Veggies

Ingredients:
- 1 cup diced butternut squash
- 1 cup diced sweet potato
- 1 cup diced bell pepper

- 1 tablespoon olive oil
- 1 tablespoon olive oil
- 1 large onion, diced
- 2 carrots, peeled and diced
- 2 celery stalks, diced
- 3 cloves garlic, minced
- 1 cup dried brown lentils, rinsed
- 6 cups vegetable broth
- 1 (15 oz) can diced tomatoes
- 2 cups chopped spinach
- 1 teaspoon dried thyme
- 1/2 teaspoon ground cumin
- 1/2 teaspoon salt
- 1/4 teaspoon ground black pepper

Nutritional Information (per serving):
- Calories: 310
- Total Fat: 6g
- Saturated Fat: 1g
- Carbohydrates: 48g
- Fiber: 13g
- Protein: 17g

Cooking Time: 55 minutes
Serving Size: 1 1/2 cups

Instructions:

1. Preheat the oven to 400°F (200°C).

2. On a baking sheet, toss the diced butternut squash, sweet potato, and bell pepper with 1 tablespoon of olive oil. Roast for 20-25 minutes, or until the vegetables are tender and slightly caramelized.

3. In a large pot or Dutch oven, heat the remaining 1 tablespoon of olive oil over medium heat.

4. Add the diced onion, carrots, and celery. Sauté for 5-7 minutes, until the vegetables are softened.

5. Stir in the minced garlic and cook for 1 minute, until fragrant.

6. Add the rinsed lentils, vegetable broth, diced tomatoes, chopped spinach, thyme, cumin, salt, and pepper.

7. Bring the soup to a boil, then reduce the heat and simmer for 25-30 minutes, or until the lentils are tender.

8. Stir in the roasted vegetables and adjust seasoning as needed.

9. Serve the soup hot, garnished with additional fresh herbs or a drizzle of olive oil, if desired.

Recipe 3:

Lentil and Vegetable Soup with Quinoa

Ingredients:
- 1 tablespoon olive oil
- 1 large onion, diced
- 3 carrots, peeled and diced
- 2 celery stalks, diced
- 4 cloves garlic, minced
- 1 cup dried green lentils, rinsed
- 1/2 cup uncooked quinoa
- 6 cups vegetable broth
- 1 (14.5 oz) can diced tomatoes
- 2 cups chopped kale
- 1 teaspoon dried thyme
- 1 teaspoon dried oregano
- 1/2 teaspoon salt
- 1/4 teaspoon ground black pepper

Nutritional Information (per serving):

- Calories: 330
- Total Fat: 6g
- Saturated Fat: 1g
- Carbohydrates: 51g
- Fiber: 14g
- Protein: 19g

Cooking Time: 50 minutes
Serving Size: 1 1/2 cups

Instructions:
1. In a large pot or Dutch oven, heat the olive oil over medium heat.
2. Add the diced onion, carrots, and celery. Sauté for 5-7 minutes, until the vegetables are softened.
3. Stir in the minced garlic and cook for 1 minute, until fragrant.
4. Add the rinsed lentils, uncooked quinoa, vegetable broth, diced tomatoes, chopped kale, thyme, oregano, salt, and pepper.
5. Bring the soup to a boil, then reduce the heat and simmer for 30-35 minutes,

or until the lentils and quinoa are tender.

6. Taste and adjust seasoning as needed.

7. Serve the soup hot, garnished with additional fresh herbs or a drizzle of olive oil, if desired.

Recipe 4:

Lentil and Vegetable Soup with Pesto Drizzle

Ingredients:
- 1 tablespoon olive oil
- 1 large onion, diced
- 3 carrots, peeled and diced
- 2 celery stalks, diced
- 3 cloves garlic, minced
- 1 cup dried red lentils, rinsed
- 6 cups vegetable broth
- 1 (15 oz) can diced tomatoes
- 2 cups chopped cauliflower
- 1 teaspoon dried basil
- 1 teaspoon dried oregano
- 1/2 teaspoon salt

- 1/4 teaspoon ground black pepper

Pesto Drizzle:
- 1/4 cup fresh basil leaves
- 2 tablespoons pine nuts
- 1 clove garlic
- 2 tablespoons olive oil
- 1 tablespoon grated Parmesan cheese
- 1 tablespoon lemon juice
- 1/4 teaspoon salt

Nutritional Information (per serving):
- Calories: 290
- Total Fat: 10g
- Saturated Fat: 2g
- Carbohydrates: 36g
- Fiber: 12g
- Protein: 16g

Cooking Time: 45 minutes
Serving Size: 1 1/2 cups soup with 1 tablespoon pesto drizzle

Instructions:

1. In a large pot or Dutch oven, heat the olive oil over medium heat.
2. Add the diced onion, carrots, and celery. Sauté for 5-7 minutes, until the vegetables are softened.
3. Stir in the minced garlic and cook for 1 minute, until fragrant.
4. Add the rinsed red lentils, vegetable broth, diced tomatoes, chopped cauliflower, basil, oregano, salt, and pepper.
5. Bring the soup to a boil, then reduce the heat and simmer for 20-25 minutes, or until the lentils are tender.
6. In a food processor, blend the ingredients for the pesto drizzle until smooth.
7. Serve the soup hot, drizzled with the pesto.

Quinoa Bowl with Roasted Veggies and Tahini Dressing

Recipe 1:

Classic Quinoa Bowl with Roasted Veggies and Tahini Dressing

Ingredients:
- 1 cup uncooked quinoa, rinsed
- 2 cups vegetable broth
- 1 cup diced sweet potato
- 1 cup diced zucchini
- 1 cup diced bell pepper
- 1 tablespoon olive oil
- 1/2 teaspoon salt
- 1/4 teaspoon ground black pepper

Tahini Dressing:
- 1/4 cup tahini
- 2 tablespoons lemon juice
- 2 tablespoons water
- 1 tablespoon maple syrup
- 1 garlic clove, minced
- 1/4 teaspoon salt
- 1/8 teaspoon ground cumin

Nutritional Information (per serving):
- Calories: 400

- Total Fat: 18g
- Saturated Fat: 2.5g
- Carbohydrates: 50g
- Fiber: 7g
- Protein: 13g

Cooking Time: 45 minutes
Serving Size: 1 1/2 cups quinoa bowl with 2 tablespoons tahini dressing

Instructions:
1. Preheat the oven to 400°F (200°C).
2. In a medium saucepan, combine the rinsed quinoa and vegetable broth. Bring to a boil, then reduce heat to low, cover, and simmer for 15-20 minutes, or until the quinoa is tender and the liquid is absorbed.
3. On a large baking sheet, toss the diced sweet potato, zucchini, and bell pepper with the olive oil, salt, and black pepper.
4. Roast the vegetables in the preheated oven for 20-25 minutes, stirring halfway, until they are tender and lightly browned.

5. In a small bowl, whisk together all the ingredients for the tahini dressing until smooth and creamy.

6. Divide the cooked quinoa among 4 bowls. Top each bowl with the roasted vegetables.

7. Drizzle the tahini dressing over the quinoa and veggies, and serve.

Recipe 2:

Quinoa Bowl with Roasted Veggies, Chickpeas, and Tahini Dressing

Ingredients:
- 1 cup uncooked quinoa, rinsed
- 2 cups vegetable broth
- 1 cup diced butternut squash
- 1 cup diced cauliflower
- 1 cup diced red onion
- 1 (15 oz) can chickpeas, drained and rinsed
- 1 tablespoon olive oil
- 1/2 teaspoon salt
- 1/4 teaspoon ground black pepper

Tahini Dressing:
- 1/3 cup tahini
- 3 tablespoons lemon juice
- 2 tablespoons water
- 1 tablespoon honey
- 1 garlic clove, minced
- 1/4 teaspoon salt
- 1/8 teaspoon ground cumin

Nutritional Information (per serving):
- Calories: 450
- Total Fat: 20g
- Saturated Fat: 3g
- Carbohydrates: 55g
- Fiber: 10g
- Protein: 15g

Cooking Time: 50 minutes
Serving Size: 1 1/2 cups quinoa bowl with 2 tablespoons tahini dressing

Instructions:
1. Preheat the oven to 400°F (200°C).

2. In a medium saucepan, combine the rinsed quinoa and vegetable broth. Bring to a boil, then reduce heat to low, cover, and simmer for 15-20 minutes, or until the quinoa is tender and the liquid is absorbed.

3. On a large baking sheet, toss the diced butternut squash, cauliflower, and red onion with the olive oil, salt, and black pepper.

4. Roast the vegetables in the preheated oven for 25-30 minutes, stirring halfway, until they are tender and lightly browned.

5. In a small bowl, whisk together all the ingredients for the tahini dressing until smooth and creamy.

6. Divide the cooked quinoa among 4 bowls. Top each bowl with the roasted vegetables and drained, rinsed chickpeas.

7. Drizzle the tahini dressing over the quinoa, veggies, and chickpeas, and serve.

Recipe 3:

Quinoa Bowl with Roasted Veggies, Avocado, and Tahini Dressing

Ingredients:
- 1 cup uncooked quinoa, rinsed
- 2 cups vegetable broth
- 1 cup diced beets
- 1 cup diced eggplant
- 1 cup diced red onion
- 1 avocado, diced
- 1 tablespoon olive oil
- 1/2 teaspoon salt
- 1/4 teaspoon ground black pepper

Tahini Dressing:
- 1/4 cup tahini
- 3 tablespoons lemon juice
- 2 tablespoons water
- 1 tablespoon maple syrup
- 1 garlic clove, minced
- 1/4 teaspoon salt
- 1/8 teaspoon ground cumin

Nutritional Information (per serving):
- Calories: 430
- Total Fat: 21g
- Saturated Fat: 3g
- Carbohydrates: 50g
- Fiber: 11g
- Protein: 12g

Cooking Time: 50 minutes
Serving Size: 1 1/2 cups quinoa bowl with 2 tablespoons tahini dressing

Instructions:
1. Preheat the oven to 400°F (200°C).
2. In a medium saucepan, combine the rinsed quinoa and vegetable broth. Bring to a boil, then reduce heat to low, cover, and simmer for 15-20 minutes, or until the quinoa is tender and the liquid is absorbed.
3. On a large baking sheet, toss the diced beets, eggplant, and red onion with the olive oil, salt, and black pepper.

4. Roast the vegetables in the preheated oven for 25-30 minutes, stirring halfway, until they are tender and lightly browned.
5. In a small bowl, whisk together all the ingredients for the tahini dressing until smooth and creamy.
6. Divide the cooked quinoa among 4 bowls. Top each bowl with the roasted vegetables and diced avocado.
7. Drizzle the tahini dressing over the quinoa, veggies, and avocado, and serve.

Recipe 4:

 Quinoa Bowl with Roasted Veggies, Feta, and Tahini Dressing

Ingredients:
- 1 cup uncooked quinoa, rinsed
- 2 cups vegetable broth
- 1 cup diced sweet potato
- 1 cup diced Brussels sprouts
- 1 cup diced red pepper
- 1/2 cup crumbled feta cheese

- 1 tablespoon olive oil
- 1/2 teaspoon salt
- 1/4 teaspoon ground black pepper

Tahini Dressing:
- 1/3 cup tahini
- 2 tablespoons lemon juice
- 2 tablespoons water
- 1 tablespoon honey
- 1 garlic clove, minced
- 1/4 teaspoon salt
- 1/8 teaspoon ground cumin

Nutritional Information (per serving):
- Calories: 440
- Total Fat: 20g
- Saturated Fat: 4g
- Carbohydrates: 50g
- Fiber: 9g
- Protein: 14g

Cooking Time: 45 minutes
Serving Size: 1 1/2 cups quinoa bowl
with 2 tablespoons tahini dressing

Instructions:
1. Preheat the oven to 400°F (200°C).
2. In a medium saucepan, combine the rinsed quinoa and vegetable broth. Bring to a boil, then reduce heat to low, cover, and simmer for 15-20 minutes, or until the quinoa is tender and the liquid is absorbed.
3. On a large baking sheet, toss the diced sweet potato, Brussels sprouts, and red pepper with the olive oil, salt, and black pepper.
4. Roast the vegetables in the preheated oven for 20-25 minutes, stirring halfway, until they are tender and lightly browned.
5. In a small bowl, whisk together all the ingredients for the tahini dressing until smooth and creamy.
6. Divide the cooked quinoa among 4 bowls. Top each bowl with the roasted vegetables and crumbled feta cheese.
7. Drizzle the tahini dressing over the quinoa, veggies, and feta, and serve.

Turkey and Veggie Wrap with Hummus

Recipe 1:

Classic Turkey and Veggie Wrap with Hummus

Ingredients:
- 4 (8-inch) whole wheat tortillas
- 8 ounces sliced turkey breast
- 1 cup shredded carrots
- 1 cup sliced cucumber
- 1 cup baby spinach leaves
- 1/2 cup hummus
- 1 tablespoon olive oil
- 1/4 teaspoon salt
- 1/8 teaspoon ground black pepper

Nutritional Information (per serving):
- Calories: 310
- Total Fat: 10g
- Saturated Fat: 1.5g
- Carbohydrates: 37g

- Fiber: 6g
- Protein: 20g

Cooking Time: 15 minutes
Serving Size: 1 wrap

Instructions:
1. Lay the tortillas on a flat surface.
2. Spread 2 tablespoons of hummus evenly over each tortilla, leaving a 1-inch border.
3. Arrange the sliced turkey, shredded carrots, sliced cucumber, and baby spinach leaves in the center of each tortilla.
4. Drizzle 1/4 teaspoon of olive oil over the veggies on each wrap, and season with a pinch of salt and pepper.
5. Fold the bottom of the tortilla up over the filling, then fold in the sides and roll up tightly to create a wrap.
6. Slice each wrap in half diagonally and serve.

Recipe 2:

Turkey and Veggie Wrap with Hummus and Avocado

Ingredients:
- 4 (8-inch) whole grain tortillas
- 8 ounces sliced turkey breast
- 1 avocado, sliced
- 1 cup cherry tomatoes, halved
- 1/2 cup sliced red onion
- 1/2 cup hummus
- 1 tablespoon olive oil
- 1/4 teaspoon salt
- 1/8 teaspoon ground black pepper

Nutritional Information (per serving):
- Calories: 380
- Total Fat: 16g
- Saturated Fat: 2.5g
- Carbohydrates: 41g
- Fiber: 8g
- Protein: 22g

Cooking Time: 20 minutes
Serving Size: 1 wrap

Instructions:
1. Lay the tortillas on a flat surface.
2. Spread 2 tablespoons of hummus evenly over each tortilla, leaving a 1-inch border.
3. Arrange the sliced turkey, avocado slices, cherry tomatoes, and sliced red onion in the center of each tortilla.
4. Drizzle 1/4 teaspoon of olive oil over the fillings on each wrap, and season with a pinch of salt and pepper.
5. Fold the bottom of the tortilla up over the filling, then fold in the sides and roll up tightly to create a wrap.
6. Slice each wrap in half diagonally and serve.

Recipe 3:

Turkey and Veggie Wrap with Hummus and Feta

Ingredients:
- 4 (8-inch) whole wheat tortillas

- 8 ounces sliced turkey breast
- 1 cup shredded red cabbage
- 1/2 cup diced bell pepper
- 1/4 cup crumbled feta cheese
- 1/2 cup hummus
- 1 tablespoon olive oil
- 1/4 teaspoon salt
- 1/8 teaspoon ground black pepper

Nutritional Information (per serving):
- Calories: 350
- Total Fat: 13g
- Saturated Fat: 3g
- Carbohydrates: 38g
- Fiber: 6g
- Protein: 23g

Cooking Time: 15 minutes
Serving Size: 1 wrap

Instructions:
1. Lay the tortillas on a flat surface.
2. Spread 2 tablespoons of hummus evenly over each tortilla, leaving a 1-inch border.

3. Arrange the sliced turkey, shredded red cabbage, diced bell pepper, and crumbled feta cheese in the center of each tortilla.
4. Drizzle 1/4 teaspoon of olive oil over the fillings on each wrap, and season with a pinch of salt and pepper.
5. Fold the bottom of the tortilla up over the filling, then fold in the sides and roll up tightly to create a wrap.
6. Slice each wrap in half diagonally and serve.

Recipe 4:

Turkey and Veggie Wrap with Hummus and Roasted Veggies

Ingredients:
- 4 (8-inch) whole grain tortillas
- 8 ounces sliced turkey breast
- 1 cup roasted sweet potato cubes
- 1 cup roasted broccoli florets
- 1/2 cup hummus
- 1 tablespoon olive oil

- 1/4 teaspoon salt
- 1/8 teaspoon ground black pepper

Nutritional Information (per serving):
- Calories: 390
- Total Fat: 12g
- Saturated Fat: 2g
- Carbohydrates: 46g
- Fiber: 8g
- Protein: 25g

Cooking Time: 30 minutes
Serving Size: 1 wrap

Instructions:
1. Preheat the oven to 400°F (200°C).
2. Toss the sweet potato cubes and broccoli florets with 1 tablespoon of olive oil, salt, and pepper. Roast for 20-25 minutes, or until tender and lightly browned.
3. Lay the tortillas on a flat surface.
4. Spread 2 tablespoons of hummus evenly over each tortilla, leaving a 1-inch border.

5. Arrange the sliced turkey, roasted sweet potato cubes, and roasted broccoli florets in the center of each tortilla.
6. Fold the bottom of the tortilla up over the filling, then fold in the sides and roll up tightly to create a wrap.
7. Slice each wrap in half diagonally and serve.

CHAPTER THREE

Dinner Recipes

Baked Chicken with Roasted Sweet Potatoes and Broccoli

Recipe 1:

Classic Baked Chicken with Roasted Sweet Potatoes and Broccoli

Ingredients:
- 4 boneless, skinless chicken breasts (about 6 oz each)
- 2 medium sweet potatoes, peeled and cubed
- 3 cups broccoli florets
- 2 tablespoons olive oil, divided
- 1 teaspoon garlic powder
- 1 teaspoon dried thyme

- 1/2 teaspoon salt
- 1/4 teaspoon ground black pepper

Nutritional Information (per serving):
- Calories: 350
- Total Fat: 9g
- Saturated Fat: 1.5g
- Carbohydrates: 29g
- Fiber: 6g
- Protein: 39g

Cooking Time: 45 minutes
Serving Size: 1 chicken breast, 1/2 cup sweet potatoes, 3/4 cup broccoli

Instructions:
1. Preheat the oven to 400°F (200°C).
2. Place the chicken breasts in a baking dish and drizzle with 1 tablespoon of olive oil. Season with garlic powder, thyme, salt, and pepper.
3. On a separate baking sheet, toss the cubed sweet potatoes and broccoli florets with the remaining 1 tablespoon

of olive oil. Season with a pinch of salt and pepper.

4. Bake the chicken and vegetables in the preheated oven for 30-35 minutes, or until the chicken is cooked through and the vegetables are tender.

5. Serve the baked chicken with the roasted sweet potatoes and broccoli.

Recipe 2:

Baked Chicken with Maple-Roasted Sweet Potatoes and Broccoli

Ingredients:
- 4 boneless, skinless chicken breasts (about 6 oz each)
- 2 medium sweet potatoes, peeled and cubed
- 3 cups broccoli florets
- 2 tablespoons olive oil, divided
- 2 tablespoons pure maple syrup
- 1 teaspoon smoked paprika
- 1/2 teaspoon salt
- 1/4 teaspoon ground black pepper

Nutritional Information (per serving):
- Calories: 370
- Total Fat: 10g
- Saturated Fat: 1.5g
- Carbohydrates: 35g
- Fiber: 6g
- Protein: 39g

Cooking Time: 45 minutes
Serving Size: 1 chicken breast, 1/2 cup sweet potatoes, 3/4 cup broccoli

Instructions:
1. Preheat the oven to 400°F (200°C).
2. Place the chicken breasts in a baking dish and drizzle with 1 tablespoon of olive oil. Season with smoked paprika, salt, and pepper.
3. On a separate baking sheet, toss the cubed sweet potatoes and broccoli florets with the remaining 1 tablespoon of olive oil and maple syrup.
4. Bake the chicken and vegetables in the preheated oven for 30-35 minutes,

or until the chicken is cooked through and the vegetables are tender.
5. Serve the baked chicken with the maple-roasted sweet potatoes and broccoli.

Recipe 3:

Baked Chicken with Parmesan-Roasted Sweet Potatoes and Broccoli

Ingredients:
- 4 boneless, skinless chicken breasts (about 6 oz each)
- 2 medium sweet potatoes, peeled and cubed
- 3 cups broccoli florets
- 2 tablespoons olive oil, divided
- 1/4 cup grated Parmesan cheese
- 1 teaspoon dried oregano
- 1/2 teaspoon salt
- 1/4 teaspoon ground black pepper

Nutritional Information (per serving):
- Calories: 380

- Total Fat: 11g
- Saturated Fat: 3g
- Carbohydrates: 31g
- Fiber: 6g
- Protein: 42g

Cooking Time: 45 minutes
Serving Size: 1 chicken breast, 1/2 cup sweet potatoes, 3/4 cup broccoli

Instructions:
1. Preheat the oven to 400°F (200°C).
2. Place the chicken breasts in a baking dish and drizzle with 1 tablespoon of olive oil. Season with salt and pepper.
3. On a separate baking sheet, toss the cubed sweet potatoes and broccoli florets with the remaining 1 tablespoon of olive oil, Parmesan cheese, and dried oregano.
4. Bake the chicken and vegetables in the preheated oven for 30-35 minutes, or until the chicken is cooked through and the vegetables are tender.

5. Serve the baked chicken with the Parmesan-roasted sweet potatoes and broccoli.

Recipe 4:

Baked Chicken with Herb-Roasted Sweet Potatoes and Broccoli

Ingredients:
- 4 boneless, skinless chicken breasts (about 6 oz each)
- 2 medium sweet potatoes, peeled and cubed
- 3 cups broccoli florets
- 2 tablespoons olive oil, divided
- 1 tablespoon chopped fresh rosemary
- 1 tablespoon chopped fresh thyme
- 1 teaspoon garlic powder
- 1/2 teaspoon salt
- 1/4 teaspoon ground black pepper

Nutritional Information (per serving):
- Calories: 360
- Total Fat: 10g

- Saturated Fat: 1.5g
- Carbohydrates: 33g
- Fiber: 7g
- Protein: 39g

Cooking Time: 45 minutes
Serving Size: 1 chicken breast, 1/2 cup sweet potatoes, 3/4 cup broccoli

Instructions:
1. Preheat the oven to 400°F (200°C).
2. Place the chicken breasts in a baking dish and drizzle with 1 tablespoon of olive oil. Season with garlic powder, salt, and pepper.
3. On a separate baking sheet, toss the cubed sweet potatoes and broccoli florets with the remaining 1 tablespoon of olive oil, chopped rosemary, and chopped thyme.
4. Bake the chicken and vegetables in the preheated oven for 30-35 minutes, or until the chicken is cooked through and the vegetables are tender.

5. Serve the baked chicken with the herb-roasted sweet potatoes and broccoli.

Blackened Tilapia with Mango Salsa and Cauliflower Rice

Recipe 1:

Blackened Tilapia with Mango Salsa and Cauliflower Rice

Ingredients:
- 4 tilapia fillets (about 6 oz each)
- 2 tbsp blackened seasoning
- 1 tbsp olive oil
- 1 mango, diced
- 1/2 red onion, diced
- 1 jalapeño, seeded and diced
- 1/4 cup chopped cilantro
- 1 tbsp lime juice
- 1 head cauliflower, riced
- Salt and pepper to taste

Nutritional Information (per serving):
- Calories: 320
- Total Fat: 12g
- Saturated Fat: 2g
- Cholesterol: 85mg
- Sodium: 680mg
- Total Carbs: 24g
- Fiber: 6g
- Sugars: 10g
- Protein: 33g

Cooking Time: 30 minutes
Servings: 4

Instructions:
1. Preheat your oven to 400°F (200°C).
2. Season the tilapia fillets evenly with the blackened seasoning.
3. Heat the olive oil in a large oven-safe skillet over medium-high heat. Add the seasoned tilapia fillets and cook for 3-4 minutes per side, until a nice crust forms.

4. Transfer the skillet to the preheated oven and bake for 8-10 minutes, or until the tilapia is cooked through.
5. In a medium bowl, combine the diced mango, red onion, jalapeño, cilantro, and lime juice. Season with salt and pepper to taste.
6. In a large microwave-safe bowl, cook the riced cauliflower in the microwave for 4-5 minutes, or until tender.
7. Serve the blackened tilapia fillets with the mango salsa and cauliflower rice.

Recipe 2:

Blackened Tilapia with Mango Salsa and Cauliflower Rice

Ingredients:
- 4 tilapia fillets (about 6 oz each)
- 2 tbsp Cajun seasoning
- 1 tbsp avocado oil
- 1 ripe mango, diced
- 1/2 cup diced red bell pepper
- 1/4 cup diced red onion

- 2 tbsp chopped fresh cilantro
- 1 tbsp lime juice
- 1 head cauliflower, riced
- Salt and pepper to taste

Nutritional Information (per serving):
- Calories: 310
- Total Fat: 13g
- Saturated Fat: 2g
- Cholesterol: 85mg
- Sodium: 610mg
- Total Carbs: 22g
- Fiber: 5g
- Sugars: 9g
- Protein: 32g

Cooking Time: 25 minutes
Servings: 4

Instructions:
1. Preheat your oven to 400°F (200°C).
2. Pat the tilapia fillets dry and season them evenly with the Cajun seasoning.
3. Heat the avocado oil in a large oven-safe skillet over medium-high heat. Add

the seasoned tilapia fillets and cook for 3-4 minutes per side, until a nice crust forms.
4. Transfer the skillet to the preheated oven and bake for 6-8 minutes, or until the tilapia is cooked through.
5. In a medium bowl, combine the diced mango, red bell pepper, red onion, cilantro, and lime juice. Season with salt and pepper to taste.
6. In a large microwave-safe bowl, cook the riced cauliflower in the microwave for 4-5 minutes, or until tender.
7. Serve the blackened tilapia fillets with the mango salsa and cauliflower rice.

Recipe 3:

Blackened Tilapia with Mango Salsa and Cauliflower Rice

Ingredients:
- 4 tilapia fillets (about 6 oz each)
- 2 tbsp blackened seasoning
- 1 tbsp coconut oil

- 1 ripe mango, diced
- 1/2 cup diced red onion
- 1 jalapeño, seeded and diced
- 2 tbsp chopped fresh cilantro
- 1 tbsp lime juice
- 1 head cauliflower, riced
- Salt and pepper to taste

Nutritional Information (per serving):
- Calories: 330
- Total Fat: 14g
- Saturated Fat: 8g
- Cholesterol: 85mg
- Sodium: 660mg
- Total Carbs: 23g
- Fiber: 6g
- Sugars: 10g
- Protein: 34g

Cooking Time: 30 minutes
Servings: 4

Instructions:
1. Preheat your oven to 400°F (200°C).

2. Coat the tilapia fillets evenly with the blackened seasoning.

3. Heat the coconut oil in a large oven-safe skillet over medium-high heat. Add the seasoned tilapia fillets and cook for 3-4 minutes per side, until a nice crust forms.

4. Transfer the skillet to the preheated oven and bake for 8-10 minutes, or until the tilapia is cooked through.

5. In a medium bowl, combine the diced mango, red onion, jalapeño, cilantro, and lime juice. Season with salt and pepper to taste.

6. In a large microwave-safe bowl, cook the riced cauliflower in the microwave for 4-5 minutes, or until tender.

7. Serve the blackened tilapia fillets with the mango salsa and cauliflower rice.

Recipe 4:

Blackened Tilapia with Mango Salsa and Cauliflower Rice

Ingredients:
- 4 tilapia fillets (about 6 oz each)
- 2 tbsp homemade blackened seasoning (blend of paprika, garlic powder, onion powder, cayenne, and salt)
- 1 tbsp grapeseed oil
- 1 ripe mango, diced
- 1/4 cup diced red onion
- 1 jalapeño, seeded and minced
- 2 tbsp chopped fresh cilantro
- 1 tbsp lime juice
- 1 head cauliflower, riced
- Salt and pepper to taste

Nutritional Information (per serving):
- Calories: 340
- Total Fat: 15g
- Saturated Fat: 2g
- Cholesterol: 90mg
- Sodium: 680mg
- Total Carbs: 25g
- Fiber: 7g
- Sugars: 11g
- Protein: 35g

Cooking Time: 35 minutes
Servings: 4

Instructions:
1. Preheat your oven to 400°F (200°C).
2. Rub the tilapia fillets evenly with the homemade blackened seasoning.
3. Heat the grapeseed oil in a large oven-safe skillet over medium-high heat. Add the seasoned tilapia fillets and cook for 3-4 minutes per side, until a nice crust forms.
4. Transfer the skillet to the preheated oven and bake for 10-12 minutes, or until the tilapia is cooked through.
5. In a medium bowl, combine the diced mango, red onion, jalapeño, cilantro, and lime juice. Season with salt and pepper to taste.
6. In a large microwave-safe bowl, cook the riced cauliflower in the microwave for 4-5 minutes, or until tender.
7. Serve the blackened tilapia fillets with the mango salsa and cauliflower rice.

Beef and Barley Stew

Recipe 1:

Beef and Barley Stew

Ingredients:
- 1 lb beef stew meat, cut into 1-inch cubes
- 2 tbsp olive oil
- 1 onion, diced
- 3 carrots, peeled and sliced
- 2 celery stalks, sliced
- 3 cloves garlic, minced
- 1 cup pearl barley
- 4 cups beef broth
- 1 (14.5 oz) can diced tomatoes
- 1 tsp dried thyme
- 1 bay leaf
- Salt and pepper to taste
- Chopped parsley for garnish (optional)

Nutritional Information (per serving):
- Calories: 350
- Total Fat: 12g

- Saturated Fat: 3g
- Cholesterol: 60mg
- Sodium: 690mg
- Total Carbs: 39g
- Fiber: 8g
- Sugars: 6g
- Protein: 27g

Cooking Time: 1 hour 30 minutes
Servings: 6

Instructions:
1. In a large Dutch oven or heavy-bottomed pot, heat the olive oil over medium-high heat.
2. Add the beef cubes and brown on all sides, about 5 minutes total. Remove the beef from the pot and set aside.
3. Add the onion, carrots, and celery to the pot. Cook for 5-7 minutes, until vegetables start to soften.
4. Add the garlic and cook for 1 minute, until fragrant.

5. Stir in the pearl barley, beef broth, diced tomatoes, thyme, and bay leaf. Return the beef to the pot.

6. Bring the stew to a boil, then reduce the heat to low, cover, and simmer for 1 to 1.5 hours, or until the beef is tender and the barley is cooked through.

7. Season with salt and pepper to taste.

8. Serve the beef and barley stew warm, garnished with chopped parsley if desired.

Recipe 2:

Beef and Barley Stew

Ingredients:
- 1.5 lbs beef chuck, cut into 1-inch cubes
- 2 tbsp all-purpose flour
- 2 tbsp vegetable oil
- 1 onion, diced
- 3 carrots, peeled and sliced
- 2 celery stalks, sliced
- 4 cloves garlic, minced
- 1 cup pearl barley

- 6 cups beef broth
- 1 (14.5 oz) can diced tomatoes
- 2 tsp Worcestershire sauce
- 1 tsp dried rosemary
- 1 bay leaf
- Salt and pepper to taste
- Chopped parsley for garnish (optional)

Nutritional Information (per serving):
- Calories: 370
- Total Fat: 14g
- Saturated Fat: 4g
- Cholesterol: 65mg
- Sodium: 790mg
- Total Carbs: 40g
- Fiber: 8g
- Sugars: 7g
- Protein: 28g

Cooking Time: 1 hour 45 minutes
Servings: 6

Instructions:
1. Pat the beef cubes dry and toss them with the flour until evenly coated.

2. Heat the vegetable oil in a large Dutch oven or heavy-bottomed pot over medium-high heat.

3. Working in batches, brown the beef cubes on all sides, about 3-4 minutes per batch. Remove the browned beef from the pot and set aside.

4. Add the onion, carrots, and celery to the pot. Cook for 5-7 minutes, until the vegetables start to soften.

5. Add the garlic and cook for 1 minute, until fragrant.

6. Stir in the pearl barley, beef broth, diced tomatoes, Worcestershire sauce, rosemary, and bay leaf. Return the browned beef to the pot.

7. Bring the stew to a boil, then reduce the heat to low, cover, and simmer for 1.5 hours, or until the beef is tender and the barley is cooked through.

8. Season with salt and pepper to taste.

9. Serve the beef and barley stew warm, garnished with chopped parsley if desired.

Recipe 3:

Beef and Barley Stew

Ingredients:
- 1.25 lbs beef stew meat, cut into 1-inch cubes
- 2 tbsp olive oil
- 1 onion, diced
- 3 carrots, peeled and sliced
- 2 celery stalks, sliced
- 4 cloves garlic, minced
- 1 cup pearl barley
- 5 cups beef broth
- 1 (15 oz) can diced tomatoes
- 2 tsp dried thyme
- 1 tsp dried rosemary
- 1 bay leaf
- Salt and pepper to taste
- Chopped parsley for garnish (optional)

Nutritional Information (per serving):
- Calories: 360
- Total Fat: 13g
- Saturated Fat: 3g

- Cholesterol: 60mg
- Sodium: 760mg
- Total Carbs: 37g
- Fiber: 8g
- Sugars: 6g
- Protein: 29g

Cooking Time: 1 hour 30 minutes
Servings: 6

Instructions:
1. In a large Dutch oven or heavy-bottomed pot, heat the olive oil over medium-high heat.
2. Add the beef cubes and brown on all sides, about 5-7 minutes total. Remove the beef from the pot and set aside.
3. Add the onion, carrots, and celery to the pot. Cook for 6-8 minutes, until the vegetables start to soften.
4. Add the garlic and cook for 1 minute, until fragrant.
5. Stir in the pearl barley, beef broth, diced tomatoes, thyme, rosemary, and

bay leaf. Return the browned beef to the pot.

6. Bring the stew to a boil, then reduce the heat to low, cover, and simmer for 1 to 1.5 hours, or until the beef is tender and the barley is cooked through.

7. Season with salt and pepper to taste.

8. Serve the beef and barley stew warm, garnished with chopped parsley if desired.

Recipe 4:

Beef and Barley Stew

Ingredients:
- 1.75 lbs beef chuck, cut into 1-inch cubes
- 2 tbsp all-purpose flour
- 3 tbsp vegetable oil
- 1 onion, diced
- 4 carrots, peeled and sliced
- 3 celery stalks, sliced
- 3 cloves garlic, minced
- 1.5 cups pearl barley

- 6 cups beef broth
- 1 (28 oz) can diced tomatoes
- 2 tsp Worcestershire sauce
- 1 tsp dried oregano
- 1 bay leaf
- Salt and pepper to taste
- Chopped parsley for garnish (optional)

Nutritional Information (per serving):
- Calories: 390
- Total Fat: 15g
- Saturated Fat: 4g
- Cholesterol: 70mg
- Sodium: 830mg
- Total Carbs: 41g
- Fiber: 9g
- Sugars: 7g
- Protein: 30g

Cooking Time: 2 hours
Servings: 6

Instructions:
1. Toss the beef cubes with the flour until evenly coated.

2. Heat the vegetable oil in a large Dutch oven or heavy-bottomed pot over medium-high heat.

3. Working in batches, brown the beef cubes on all sides, about 4-5 minutes per batch. Remove the browned beef from the pot and set aside.

4. Add the onion, carrots, and celery to the pot. Cook for 6-8 minutes, until the vegetables start to soften.

5. Add the garlic and cook for 1 minute, until fragrant.

6. Stir in the pearl barley, beef broth, diced tomatoes, Worcestershire sauce, oregano, and bay leaf. Return the browned beef to the pot.

7. Bring the stew to a boil, then reduce the heat to low, cover, and simmer for 2 hours, or until the beef is very tender and the barley is cooked through.

8. Season with salt and pepper to taste.

9. Serve the beef and barley stew warm, garnished with chopped parsley if desired.

Vegetable Stir-Fry with Brown Rice

Recipe 1:

Vegetable Stir-Fry with Brown Rice

Ingredients:
- 1 cup uncooked brown rice
- 2 tbsp sesame oil
- 2 cloves garlic, minced
- 1 inch ginger, grated
- 1 red bell pepper, sliced
- 1 cup broccoli florets
- 1 cup sliced mushrooms
- 1 cup snow peas
- 1 cup shredded carrots
- 2 tbsp low-sodium soy sauce
- 1 tsp sesame seeds
- Salt and pepper to taste

Nutritional Information (per serving):
- Calories: 320
- Total Fat: 9g
- Saturated Fat: 1g

- Cholesterol: 0mg
- Sodium: 430mg
- Total Carbs: 50g
- Fiber: 6g
- Sugars: 4g
- Protein: 8g

Cooking Time: 30 minutes
Servings: 4

Instructions:
1. Cook the brown rice according to package instructions.
2. In a large wok or skillet, heat the sesame oil over medium-high heat.
3. Add the garlic and ginger and cook for 1 minute, until fragrant.
4. Add the bell pepper, broccoli, mushrooms, snow peas, and carrots. Stir-fry for 5-7 minutes, until the vegetables are tender-crisp.
5. Add the cooked brown rice and soy sauce. Toss everything together until well combined.

6. Sprinkle the sesame seeds over the top and season with salt and pepper to taste.

7. Serve the vegetable stir-fry with brown rice immediately.

Recipe 2:

Vegetable Stir-Fry with Brown Rice

Ingredients:
- 1.5 cups uncooked brown rice
- 2 tbsp vegetable oil
- 1 onion, sliced
- 3 cloves garlic, minced
- 1 inch ginger, grated
- 1 red bell pepper, sliced
- 1 cup sliced zucchini
- 1 cup chopped broccoli
- 1 cup sliced mushrooms
- 2 tbsp low-sodium soy sauce
- 1 tbsp rice vinegar
- 1 tsp sesame oil
- Salt and pepper to taste

- Chopped green onions for garnish (optional)

Nutritional Information (per serving):
- Calories: 350
- Total Fat: 10g
- Saturated Fat: 1g
- Cholesterol: 0mg
- Sodium: 510mg
- Total Carbs: 55g
- Fiber: 7g
- Sugars: 3g
- Protein: 9g

Cooking Time: 35 minutes
Servings: 4

Instructions:
1. Cook the brown rice according to package instructions.
2. In a large wok or skillet, heat the vegetable oil over medium-high heat.
3. Add the onion, garlic, and ginger. Cook for 2-3 minutes, until fragrant.

4. Add the bell pepper, zucchini, broccoli, and mushrooms. Stir-fry for 5-7 minutes, until the vegetables are tender-crisp.
5. Add the cooked brown rice, soy sauce, rice vinegar, and sesame oil. Toss everything together until well combined.
6. Season with salt and pepper to taste.
7. Serve the vegetable stir-fry with brown rice, garnished with chopped green onions if desired.

Recipe 3:

Vegetable Stir-Fry with Brown Rice

Ingredients:
- 1 cup uncooked brown rice
- 2 tbsp olive oil
- 1 onion, diced
- 2 carrots, sliced
- 1 cup broccoli florets
- 1 cup snow peas
- 1 cup sliced mushrooms
- 2 cloves garlic, minced

- 1 tbsp grated ginger
- 2 tbsp low-sodium soy sauce
- 1 tbsp rice vinegar
- 1 tsp sesame seeds
- Salt and pepper to taste

Nutritional Information (per serving):
- Calories: 330
- Total Fat: 11g
- Saturated Fat: 1.5g
- Cholesterol: 0mg
- Sodium: 460mg
- Total Carbs: 50g
- Fiber: 6g
- Sugars: 4g
- Protein: 9g

Cooking Time: 40 minutes
Servings: 4

Instructions:
1. Cook the brown rice according to package instructions.
2. In a large wok or skillet, heat the olive oil over medium-high heat.

3. Add the onion and cook for 2-3 minutes, until translucent.

4. Add the carrots, broccoli, snow peas, and mushrooms. Stir-fry for 5-7 minutes, until the vegetables are tender-crisp.

5. Add the garlic and ginger and cook for 1 minute, until fragrant.

6. Stir in the cooked brown rice, soy sauce, and rice vinegar. Toss everything together until well combined.

7. Sprinkle the sesame seeds over the top and season with salt and pepper to taste.

8. Serve the vegetable stir-fry with brown rice immediately.

Recipe 4:

Vegetable Stir-Fry with Brown Rice

Ingredients:
- 1.5 cups uncooked brown rice
- 2 tbsp sesame oil
- 1 red onion, sliced

- 1 red bell pepper, sliced
- 1 cup sliced shiitake mushrooms
- 1 cup snap peas
- 1 cup shredded cabbage
- 2 cloves garlic, minced
- 1 tbsp grated ginger
- 2 tbsp low-sodium soy sauce
- 1 tbsp rice vinegar
- 1 tsp sesame seeds
- Salt and pepper to taste
- Chopped cilantro for garnish (optional)

Nutritional Information (per serving):
- Calories: 360
- Total Fat: 10g
- Saturated Fat: 1.5g
- Cholesterol: 0mg
- Sodium: 540mg
- Total Carbs: 58g
- Fiber: 7g
- Sugars: 4g
- Protein: 9g

Cooking Time: 45 minutes
Servings: 4

Instructions:

1. Cook the brown rice according to package instructions.

2. In a large wok or skillet, heat the sesame oil over medium-high heat.

3. Add the red onion and bell pepper. Stir-fry for 3-4 minutes, until slightly softened.

4. Add the mushrooms, snap peas, and cabbage. Stir-fry for another 4-5 minutes, until the vegetables are tender-crisp.

5. Add the garlic and ginger. Cook for 1 minute, until fragrant.

6. Stir in the cooked brown rice, soy sauce, and rice vinegar. Toss everything together until well combined.

7. Sprinkle the sesame seeds over the top and season with salt and pepper to taste.

8. Serve the vegetable stir-fry with brown rice, garnished with chopped cilantro if desired.

CONCLUSION

As you've discovered throughout this comprehensive cookbook, eating well while managing congestive heart failure is not only possible, but can be truly delightful. The recipes showcased within these pages offer a delicious and nutritious path forward, empowering you to take an active role in your health and wellness.

Through the thoughtfully curated selection of heart-healthy meals, you'll find a renewed sense of joy and satisfaction in the kitchen. Each dish has been meticulously crafted to support your cardiovascular needs, focusing on ingredients that are low in sodium, saturated fat, and cholesterol, while still delivering an abundance of flavor. From savory main courses to nourishing soups, satisfying sides, and even indulgent desserts, this cookbook has everything you need to seamlessly incorporate heart-smart eating into your daily life.

Beyond the recipes, you'll also discover a wealth of practical information to guide you through the complexities of congestive heart failure. Expert insights on dietary guidelines, portion control, and meal planning equip you with the knowledge and tools to make informed decisions about your diet. By understanding how specific nutrients and cooking methods can impact your condition, you'll be able to tailor your meals to your unique needs, ensuring optimal heart health and overall well-being.

Embracing a heart-healthy lifestyle can seem daunting at first, but with "The Ultimate Congestive Heart Failure

Cookbook" as your trusted companion, you'll embark on a culinary journey that nourishes both your body and spirit. Prepare to rediscover the joys of eating, savor the flavors of wholesome ingredients, and ultimately, empower yourself to take charge of your health, one delicious bite at a time.

9 798333 352163

Table of Contents

Introduction 9

Understanding Dysphagia 9

Types of Dysphagia 9

Symptoms of Dysphagia 10

Diagnosis and Treatment 11

Importance of Nutrition for Seniors 12

Key Nutritional Needs for Seniors 12

Challenges in Senior Nutrition 14

Strategies for Improving Senior Nutrition 14

Essential Kitchen Tools 15

Key Ingredients for Soft Food Diets 18

Tips for Preparing Soft Foods 21

DYSPHAGIA RECIPES 23

Breakfast Ideas for Easy Swallowing 23

Creamy Oatmeal with Mashed Bananas .. 23

Smooth Apple Cinnamon Rice Porridge .. 26

Velvety Vanilla Quinoa Pudding 29

Soft Polenta with Warm Berries............... 31

Silky Pumpkin Spice Farina 33

Fluffy Scrambled Eggs with Cream Cheese 35

Soft Poached Eggs on Pureed Avocado 37

Mild Cheddar Egg Custard 40

Creamy Spinach and Egg Soufflé 42

Gentle Egg and Cheese Strata 45

Nutritious Lunches 48

Creamy Carrot Ginger Soup 48

Pureed Chicken and Vegetable Stew 51

Smooth Butternut Squash and Apple Soup 54

Silky Lentil and Spinach Stew 57

Savory Salmon Mousse 60

Soft Scrambled Eggs with Cheese 62

Tender Braised Beef Puree 64

Creamy Chicken and Broccoli Casserole ...67

Velvety Sweet Potato Puree 70

Smooth Cauliflower and Leek Mash..........72

Delicious Dinners...74

Creamy Chicken and Vegetable Puree.......74

Savory Beef and Mushroom Puree 76

Butternut Squash and Carrot Puree 78

Lentil and Spinach Puree 80

Cheesy Chicken and Broccoli Bake........... 82

Soft Tuna Noodle Casserole 84

Mild Beef and Vegetable Shepherd's Pie .. 86

Creamy Potato and Leek Bake.................. 88

Smooth Salmon and Sweet Potato Puree . 90

Creamy Cod and Spinach Puree 92

Snacks and Small Bites 95

Soft Avocado and Banana Bites............... 95

Mini Quinoa Patties................................. 96

Sweet Potato and Carrot Fritters.............. 98

Creamy Spinach and Artichoke Dip 100

Silky Hummus 102

Smooth Avocado Yogurt Dip 104

Soft Cinnamon Applesauce Bites 105

Creamy Banana Pudding.........................106

Peanut Butter Mousse 108

Soft Blueberry Muffins 110

Hydration and Desserts 112

Creamy Banana and Avocado Smoothie . 112

Blueberry Greek Yogurt Smoothie 114

Peach and Almond Milk Smoothie.......... 116

Protein-Packed Peanut Butter and Chocolate Shake 118

Soft Baked Apple Cinnamon Crumble.....120

Creamy Cheesecake Cups 122

Vanilla Bean Pudding 124

Fruit-Infused Gelatin 126

Chocolate Avocado Pudding....................128

Moist Carrot Cake with Cream Cheese Frosting 130

Introduction

Understanding Dysphagia

Dysphagia refers to difficulty swallowing and can be a significant health concern, particularly among seniors. It can result from various conditions, including neurological disorders, stroke, head or neck injuries, cancer, or age-related changes in muscle strength and coordination.

Types of Dysphagia

1. Oropharyngeal Dysphagia: Involves difficulty initiating a swallow due to problems in the mouth or throat. Causes include neurological disorders like Parkinson's disease, multiple sclerosis, or stroke.

2. Esophageal Dysphagia: Involves the sensation of food sticking or getting hung up in the base of the throat or chest after you've started to swallow. Causes include esophageal stricture, tumors, or gastroesophageal reflux disease (GERD).

Symptoms of Dysphagia

- Coughing or choking when eating or drinking
- A sensation of food being stuck in the throat or chest
- Drooling
- Hoarseness
- Regurgitation
- Unintentional weight loss
- Frequent heartburn

- Complications of Dysphagia
- Malnutrition and dehydration
- Aspiration pneumonia, caused by food or liquid entering the lungs
- Reduced quality of life

Diagnosis and Treatment

Diagnosis typically involves a physical examination, imaging tests such as X-rays or endoscopy, and functional tests like a swallowing study. Treatment depends on the underlying cause and severity. It may include swallowing therapy, dietary changes, medication, or surgery.

Importance of Nutrition for Seniors

Nutrition plays a crucial role in maintaining health and well-being, especially for seniors. Proper nutrition can help prevent or manage chronic diseases, improve immune function, and enhance quality of life.

Key Nutritional Needs for Seniors

- Protein: Essential for maintaining muscle mass and repairing tissues. Sources include lean meats, fish, eggs, dairy products, beans, and nuts.
- Fiber: Important for digestive health and preventing constipation. Sources include fruits, vegetables, whole grains, and legumes.

- Calcium and Vitamin D: Vital for bone health to prevent osteoporosis. Sources include dairy products, fortified foods, leafy green vegetables, and sunlight for vitamin D synthesis.

- Vitamin B12: Important for nerve function and red blood cell production. Sources include meat, fish, dairy, and fortified cereals.

- Hydration: Seniors are at risk of dehydration due to reduced thirst sensation. Encouraging regular fluid intake is essential.

Challenges in Senior Nutrition

1. Appetite Loss: Aging can lead to decreased appetite, affecting food intake.
2. Dental Issues: Problems with teeth or dentures can make chewing difficult.
3. Chronic Conditions: Diseases like diabetes or heart disease require specific dietary adjustments.
4. Medication Interactions: Some medications can affect appetite or nutrient absorption.

Strategies for Improving Senior Nutrition

1. Encouraging small, frequent meals rich in nutrients.
2. Making meals visually appealing and flavorful to stimulate appetite.

3. Using nutritional supplements if necessary.

4. Ensuring meals are easy to chew and swallow, especially for those with dental issues or dysphagia.

5. Essential Kitchen Tools and Equipment

6. Having the right kitchen tools and equipment is vital for preparing healthy, safe, and enjoyable meals. For seniors, tools that promote ease of use and safety are particularly important.

Essential Kitchen Tools

1. Blender or Food Processor: Crucial for making pureed foods, smoothies, and soups, especially important for those on a soft food diet due to dysphagia.

2. Microwave: Useful for quickly reheating meals and making cooking more accessible for seniors.

3. Non-Slip Cutting Board: Ensures stability while cutting and reduces the risk of accidents.

4. Sharp Knives: Sharp, easy-to-handle knives make chopping and slicing easier and safer.

5. Adaptive Utensils: Ergonomically designed utensils can help those with arthritis or limited hand strength.

6. Slow Cooker or Instant Pot: Ideal for preparing nutritious, one-pot meals with minimal effort.

7. Measuring Cups and Spoons: Ensures accurate portion control and helps in following recipes correctly.

8. Grip Mats: Placed under bowls or cutting boards to prevent slipping.

9. Jar Opener: Helps seniors open jars and bottles without straining their hands.

10. Electric Can Opener: Easier to use than manual versions, especially for those with limited hand strength.

Key Ingredients for Soft Food Diets

Soft food diets are essential for individuals with chewing or swallowing difficulties, such as those with dysphagia. These diets focus on foods that are easy to chew and swallow while still providing necessary nutrients.

Key Ingredients

Protein Sources

- Eggs: Soft-cooked eggs like scrambled or poached are easy to eat.
- Fish: Tender fish like salmon or cod, which can be easily flaked.
- Ground Meats: Ground chicken, turkey, or beef, preferably prepared as meatballs or in sauces.
- Tofu: Soft and versatile, it can be blended into smoothies or used in soups.

Dairy Products

- Yogurt: Smooth and creamy, high in protein and probiotics.
- Cheese: Soft cheeses like cottage cheese or ricotta.
- Milk: Can be used in smoothies, soups, or as a base for creamy dishes.

Fruits

- Bananas: Naturally soft and easy to mash.
- Avocado: Smooth and creamy, rich in healthy fats.
- Applesauce: Pureed apples, providing fiber and vitamin C.
- Peaches and Pears: Canned in juice, easily mashable.

Vegetables

- Mashed Potatoes: Soft and easy to eat, can be enriched with milk or cream.
- Steamed or Pureed Vegetables: Carrots, squash, and peas.
- Spinach: Cooked and finely chopped or pureed.

Grains

- Oatmeal: Soft and easy to swallow, can be enriched with milk and fruit.
- Rice: Soft-cooked rice or rice pudding.
- Pasta: Well-cooked, soft pasta in sauces or soups.

Legumes

- Lentils: Cooked until soft, can be pureed into soups.
- Beans: Well-cooked and mashed or pureed, like black beans or chickpeas.

Soups and Stews

- Broth-based Soups: With finely chopped or pureed ingredients.
- Creamy Soups: Like tomato, butternut squash, or potato leek soup.

Tips for Preparing Soft Foods

1. Blending and Pureeing: Use a blender or food processor to achieve the desired texture.
2. Cooking Methods: Steaming, boiling, or slow-cooking to ensure softness.
3. Moistening Agents: Use broth, gravy, or sauces to moisten dry foods and make them easier to swallow.
4. Seasoning: Enhance flavor with herbs and spices without adding texture.

5. Safety: Ensure foods are cooled to a safe
   temperature to prevent burns.

DYSPHAGIA RECIPES

Breakfast Ideas for Easy Swallowing

Creamy Oatmeal with Mashed Bananas

Servings: 2

Total Prep Time: 15 minutes

Ingredients:

- 1 cup rolled oats
- 2 cups milk (or water)
- 1 ripe banana, mashed
- 1 tablespoon honey or maple syrup (optional)
- 1/2 teaspoon ground cinnamon
- Pinch of salt

Directions:

1. In a medium saucepan, bring the milk (or water) to a boil.
2. Stir in the oats, reduce the heat to medium, and cook for about 5 minutes, stirring occasionally.
3. Add the mashed banana, honey or maple syrup (if using), cinnamon, and salt. Stir well to combine.
4. Continue cooking for another 2-3 minutes, or until the oatmeal reaches your desired consistency.
5. Serve hot, optionally topped with additional banana slices or a sprinkle of cinnamon.

Nutritional Info (per serving):

Calories: 220

Protein: 7g

Carbohydrates: 40g

Fiber: 4g

Sugars: 12g

Fat: 4g

Saturated Fat: 1.5g

Sodium: 60mg

Smooth Apple Cinnamon Rice Porridge

Servings: 2

Total Prep Time: 25 minutes

Ingredients:

- 1/2 cup white rice
- 2 cups water
- 1 cup milk
- 1 apple, peeled and grated
- 1 tablespoon honey or brown sugar
- 1 teaspoon ground cinnamon
- Pinch of salt

Directions:

1. In a medium saucepan, bring the water to a boil.

2. Add the rice, reduce the heat to low, and cover. Simmer for about 15 minutes or until the rice is tender.

3. Stir in the milk, grated apple, honey or brown sugar, cinnamon, and salt.

4. Cook over low heat, stirring frequently, until the porridge is creamy and thick, about 10 minutes.

5. Serve warm, optionally garnished with extra cinnamon or apple slices.

Nutritional Info (per serving):

Calories: 230

Protein: 6g

Carbohydrates: 45g

Fiber: 2g

Sugars: 18g

Fat: 3g

Saturated Fat: 1.5g

Sodium: 55mg

Velvety Vanilla Quinoa Pudding

Servings: 2

Total Prep Time: 25 minutes

Ingredients:

- 1/2 cup quinoa
- 1 cup water
- 1 cup milk
- 2 tablespoons sugar
- 1 teaspoon vanilla extract
- Pinch of salt

Directions:

1. Rinse the quinoa under cold water.
2. In a medium saucepan, bring the water to a boil. Add the quinoa, reduce the heat to low, cover, and simmer for about 15 minutes, or until the quinoa is tender and water is absorbed.

3. Stir in the milk, sugar, vanilla extract, and salt.

4. Cook over low heat, stirring frequently, until the mixture thickens to a pudding-like consistency, about 10 minutes.

5. Serve warm or chilled, optionally topped with fresh fruit or a sprinkle of cinnamon.

Nutritional Info (per serving):

Calories: 250

Protein: 8g

Carbohydrates: 40g

Fiber: 3g

Sugars: 15g

Fat: 6g

Saturated Fat: 3g

Sodium: 50mg

Soft Polenta with Warm Berries

Servings: 2

Total Prep Time: 20 minutes

Ingredients:

- 1/2 cup polenta (cornmeal)
- 2 cups water
- 1 tablespoon butter
- 1 tablespoon honey
- 1 cup mixed berries (fresh or frozen)
- 1 tablespoon sugar (optional)
- Pinch of salt

Directions:

1. In a medium saucepan, bring the water to a boil with a pinch of salt.
2. Gradually whisk in the polenta, reduce the heat to low, and cook, stirring frequently, until thick and creamy, about 15 minutes.

3. Stir in the butter and honey.

4. While the polenta cooks, warm the berries in a small saucepan over low heat, adding sugar if desired.

5. Serve the polenta topped with warm berries.

Nutritional Info (per serving):

Calories: 220

Protein: 4g

Carbohydrates: 40g

Fiber: 4g

Sugars: 18g

Fat: 6g

Saturated Fat: 3.5g

Sodium: 60mg

Silky Pumpkin Spice Farina

Servings: 2

Total Prep Time: 15 minutes

Ingredients:

- 1/2 cup farina (cream of wheat)
- 2 cups milk
- 1/2 cup canned pumpkin puree
- 2 tablespoons brown sugar
- 1 teaspoon pumpkin pie spice
- Pinch of salt

Directions:

1. In a medium saucepan, bring the milk to a boil.
2. Gradually whisk in the farina, reduce the heat to low, and cook, stirring frequently, until thickened, about 5 minutes.
3. Stir in the pumpkin puree, brown sugar, pumpkin pie spice, and salt.

4. Cook for an additional 2-3 minutes, until everything is well combined and heated through.

5. Serve warm, optionally topped with a sprinkle of cinnamon or a dollop of whipped cream.

Nutritional Info (per serving):

Calories: 240

Protein: 7g

Carbohydrates: 42g

Fiber: 3g

Sugars: 20g

Fat: 5g

Saturated Fat: 2.5g

Sodium: 55mg

Fluffy Scrambled Eggs with Cream Cheese

Servings: 2

Total Prep Time: 10 minutes

Ingredients:

- 4 large eggs
- 2 tablespoons milk or cream
- 2 tablespoons cream cheese, softened
- 1 tablespoon butter
- Salt and pepper to taste

Directions:

1. In a bowl, whisk together the eggs, milk or cream, salt, and pepper.
2. Heat the butter in a non-stick skillet over medium-low heat.

3. Pour the egg mixture into the skillet. As the eggs begin to set, add the cream cheese in small dollops.
4. Gently stir and fold the eggs until they are just cooked and the cream cheese is melted.
5. Serve immediately.

Nutritional Info (per serving):

Calories: 210

Protein: 12g

Carbohydrates: 2g

Fiber: 0g

Sugars: 1g

Fat: 18g

Saturated Fat: 9g

Sodium: 170mg

Soft Poached Eggs on Pureed Avocado

Servings: 2

Total Prep Time: 15 minutes

Ingredients:

- 4 large eggs
- 1 ripe avocado
- 1 tablespoon lemon juice
- Salt and pepper to taste
- 2 slices whole-grain bread (optional)

Directions:

1. Bring a medium pot of water to a gentle simmer. Add a splash of vinegar if desired.
2. Crack the eggs one at a time into a small bowl, then gently slide them into the simmering water. Poach for about 3-4

minutes, until the whites are set but the yolks are still runny.

3. Meanwhile, mash the avocado with lemon juice, salt, and pepper.
4. Spread the avocado puree on the toast slices (if using).
5. Remove the poached eggs with a slotted spoon and place them on top of the avocado.
6. Serve immediately.

Nutritional Info (per serving):

Calories: 250

Protein: 12g

Carbohydrates: 10g

Fiber: 5g

Sugars: 1g

Fat: 20g

Saturated Fat: 4g

Sodium: 150mg

Mild Cheddar Egg Custard

Servings: 2

Total Prep Time: 35 minutes

Ingredients:

- 2 large eggs
- 1 cup milk
- 1/2 cup shredded mild cheddar cheese
- 1/2 teaspoon salt
- 1/4 teaspoon ground white pepper
- Pinch of nutmeg

Directions:

1. Preheat the oven to 325°F (165°C). Grease two small custard cups or ramekins.
2. In a bowl, whisk together the eggs, milk, salt, pepper, and nutmeg.
3. Stir in the shredded cheddar cheese.

4. Pour the mixture into the prepared custard cups.

5. Place the cups in a baking dish and add hot water to the dish until it reaches halfway up the sides of the cups.

6. Bake for about 30 minutes, or until the custard is set and lightly golden on top.

7. Serve warm.

Nutritional Info (per serving):

Calories: 220

Protein: 14g

Carbohydrates: 5g

Fiber: 0g

Sugars: 4g

Fat: 16g

Saturated Fat: 8g

Sodium: 360mg

Creamy Spinach and Egg Soufflé

Servings: 2

Total Prep Time: 40 minutes

Ingredients:

- 3 large eggs, separated
- 1/2 cup milk
- 1/2 cup cooked spinach, finely chopped
- 1/4 cup grated Parmesan cheese
- 2 tablespoons butter
- 2 tablespoons all-purpose flour
- Salt and pepper to taste
- Pinch of nutmeg

Directions:

1. Preheat the oven to 375°F (190°C). Grease two small soufflé dishes or ramekins.

2. In a medium saucepan, melt the butter over medium heat. Stir in the flour and cook for 1-2 minutes.

3. Gradually whisk in the milk and cook, stirring constantly, until thickened.

4. Remove from heat and stir in the chopped spinach, Parmesan cheese, salt, pepper, and nutmeg.

5. Beat the egg yolks and stir them into the spinach mixture.

6. In a clean bowl, beat the egg whites until stiff peaks form. Gently fold them into the spinach mixture.

7. Divide the mixture between the prepared soufflé dishes.

8. Bake for about 20-25 minutes, or until puffed and golden.

9. Serve immediately.

Nutritional Info (per serving):

Calories: 220

Protein: 13g

Carbohydrates: 8g

Fiber: 1g

Sugars: 2g

Fat: 16g

Saturated Fat: 9g

Sodium: 340mg

Gentle Egg and Cheese Strata

Servings: 2

Total Prep Time: 1 hour (including baking time)

Ingredients:

- 4 large eggs
- 1 cup milk
- 2 cups cubed bread (preferably day-old)
- 1/2 cup shredded cheese (cheddar, mozzarella, or your choice)
- 1/4 cup finely chopped onion (optional)
- 1 tablespoon butter
- Salt and pepper to taste

Directions:

1. Preheat the oven to 350°F (175°C). Grease a small baking dish.
2. In a bowl, whisk together the eggs, milk, salt, and pepper.

3. In the prepared baking dish, layer the bread cubes, shredded cheese, and chopped onion.
4. Pour the egg mixture over the top, pressing down lightly to ensure the bread absorbs the liquid.
5. Dot with butter.
6. Bake for about 40-45 minutes, or until the strata is puffed and golden brown.
7. Let cool slightly before serving.

Nutritional Info (per serving):

Calories: 320

Protein: 17g

Carbohydrates: 22g

Fiber: 2g

Sugars: 5g

Fat: 20g

Saturated Fat: 10g

Sodium: 470mg

Nutritious Lunches

Creamy Carrot Ginger Soup

Servings: 4

Total Prep Time: 40 minutes

Ingredients:

- 1 lb carrots, peeled and chopped
- 1 large onion, chopped
- 2 tbsp fresh ginger, grated
- 3 cups vegetable broth
- 1 cup coconut milk
- 2 tbsp olive oil
- Salt and pepper to taste

Directions:

1. Heat olive oil in a large pot over medium heat.
2. Add onion and cook until softened, about 5 minutes.

3. Add ginger and cook for 1 minute until fragrant.
4. Add carrots and vegetable broth. Bring to a boil, then reduce heat and simmer for 20 minutes, until carrots are tender.
5. Puree the soup using an immersion blender or in batches in a blender until smooth.
6. Stir in coconut milk and season with salt and pepper.
7. Serve hot, garnished with fresh herbs if desired.

Nutritional Info (per serving):

Calories: 200

Protein: 3g

Fat: 14g

Carbohydrates: 18g

Fiber: 4g

Sugar: 8g

Sodium: 500mg

Pureed Chicken and Vegetable Stew

Servings: 6

Total Prep Time: 50 minutes

Ingredients:

- 1 lb chicken breast, cooked and chopped
- 2 carrots, peeled and chopped
- 2 potatoes, peeled and chopped
- 1 onion, chopped
- 2 stalks celery, chopped
- 4 cups chicken broth
- 1 cup heavy cream
- 2 tbsp olive oil
- Salt and pepper to taste

Directions:

1. Heat olive oil in a large pot over medium heat.

2. Add onion, carrots, celery, and potatoes. Cook until vegetables are softened, about 10 minutes.
3. Add chicken broth and bring to a boil. Reduce heat and simmer for 20 minutes, until vegetables are tender.
4. Add cooked chicken and cook for an additional 10 minutes.
5. Puree the stew using an immersion blender or in batches in a blender until smooth.
6. Stir in heavy cream and season with salt and pepper.
7. Serve warm.

Nutritional Info (per serving):

Calories: 280

Protein: 20g

Fat: 16g

Carbohydrates: 16g

Fiber: 3g

Sugar: 4g

Sodium: 700mg

Smooth Butternut Squash and Apple Soup

Servings: 4

Total Prep Time: 45 minutes

Ingredients:

- 1 medium butternut squash, peeled and cubed
- 2 apples, peeled and chopped
- 1 onion, chopped
- 3 cups vegetable broth
- 1 cup apple cider
- 2 tbsp olive oil
- 1 tsp ground cinnamon
- Salt and pepper to taste

Directions:

1. Heat olive oil in a large pot over medium heat.

2. Add onion and cook until softened, about 5 minutes.

3. Add butternut squash and apples, and cook for another 5 minutes.

4. Pour in vegetable broth and apple cider. Bring to a boil, then reduce heat and simmer for 20 minutes, until squash and apples are tender.

5. Puree the soup using an immersion blender or in batches in a blender until smooth.

6. Stir in cinnamon and season with salt and pepper.

7. Serve hot, garnished with a sprinkle of cinnamon if desired.

Nutritional Info (per serving):

Calories: 180

Protein: 2g

Fat: 7g

Carbohydrates: 30g

Fiber: 5g

Sugar: 15g

Sodium: 400mg

Silky Lentil and Spinach Stew

Servings: 4

Total Prep Time: 1 hour

Ingredients:

- 1 cup dried lentils, rinsed
- 2 cups fresh spinach, chopped
- 1 onion, chopped
- 2 cloves garlic, minced
- 4 cups vegetable broth
- 1 cup diced tomatoes
- 2 tbsp olive oil
- 1 tsp ground cumin
- 1 tsp ground coriander
- Salt and pepper to taste

Directions:

1. Heat olive oil in a large pot over medium heat.

2. Add onion and garlic, cooking until softened, about 5 minutes.

3. Stir in cumin and coriander, cooking until fragrant, about 1 minute.

4. Add lentils, vegetable broth, and diced tomatoes. Bring to a boil, then reduce heat and simmer for 30 minutes, until lentils are tender.

5. Add chopped spinach and cook until wilted, about 5 minutes.

6. Puree the stew using an immersion blender or in batches in a blender until smooth.

7. Season with salt and pepper.

8. Serve warm.

Nutritional Info (per serving):

Calories: 220

Protein: 12g

Fat: 7g

Carbohydrates: 30g

Fiber: 12g

Sugar: 7g

Sodium: 600mg

Savory Salmon Mousse

Servings: 6

Total Prep Time: 20 minutes (plus chilling time)

Ingredients:

- 8 oz smoked salmon
- 1 cup cream cheese, softened
- 1/2 cup heavy cream
- 1 tbsp lemon juice
- 1 tsp fresh dill, chopped
- Salt and pepper to taste

Directions:

1. In a food processor, blend smoked salmon until smooth.
2. Add cream cheese, heavy cream, lemon juice, and dill. Blend until fully combined and smooth.
3. Season with salt and pepper.

4. Transfer the mousse to a serving dish and refrigerate for at least 2 hours before serving.

5. Serve chilled, with crackers or bread.

Nutritional Info (per serving):

Calories: 220

Protein: 10g

Fat: 20g

Carbohydrates: 2g

Fiber: 0g

Sugar: 1g

Sodium: 400mg

Soft Scrambled Eggs with Cheese

Servings: 2

Total Prep Time: 10 minutes

Ingredients:

- 4 large eggs
- 1/4 cup milk
- 1/2 cup shredded cheese (cheddar or your choice)
- 2 tbsp butter
- Salt and pepper to taste

Directions:

1. In a bowl, whisk together eggs and milk until well combined.
2. Melt butter in a non-stick skillet over medium-low heat.
3. Pour in the egg mixture and let it sit undisturbed for a few seconds.

4. Stir gently, pushing the eggs from one side of the skillet to the other, until curds form.

5. When the eggs are nearly set, add the shredded cheese and continue to cook until cheese is melted and eggs are creamy.

6. Season with salt and pepper.

7. Serve immediately.

Nutritional Info (per serving):

Calories: 280

Protein: 18g

Fat: 22g

Carbohydrates: 3g

Fiber: 0g

Sugar: 2g

Sodium: 350mg

Tender Braised Beef Puree

Servings: 4

Total Prep Time: 3 hours

Ingredients:

- 1 lb beef chuck roast, cut into cubes
- 1 onion, chopped
- 2 carrots, peeled and chopped
- 2 cloves garlic, minced
- 2 cups beef broth
- 1 cup red wine (optional)
- 2 tbsp olive oil
- 1 tsp thyme
- Salt and pepper to taste

Directions:

1. Preheat oven to 300°F (150°C).
2. Heat olive oil in a large oven-safe pot over medium heat.

3. Brown beef cubes on all sides, then remove from the pot.

4. Add onion, carrots, and garlic to the pot, cooking until softened.

5. Return beef to the pot and add beef broth, red wine (if using), and thyme.

6. Bring to a boil, then cover and transfer to the oven.

7. Braise in the oven for 2.5 hours, until beef is very tender.

8. Puree the mixture using an immersion blender or in batches in a blender until smooth.

9. Season with salt and pepper.

10. Serve warm.

Nutritional Info (per serving):

Calories: 350

Protein: 28g

Fat: 20g

Carbohydrates: 8g

Fiber: 2g

Sugar: 3g

Sodium: 500mg

Creamy Chicken and Broccoli Casserole

Servings: 6

Total Prep Time: 1 hour

Ingredients:

- 1 lb chicken breast, cooked and shredded
- 3 cups broccoli florets, steamed
- 1 cup cheddar cheese, shredded
- 1 cup mozzarella cheese, shredded
- 1 cup heavy cream
- 1 cup chicken broth
- 2 cloves garlic, minced
- 1 tsp dried thyme
- Salt and pepper to taste
- 2 tbsp butter
- 2 tbsp all-purpose flour

Directions:

1. Preheat your oven to 350°F (175°C). Grease a baking dish with butter or non-stick spray.

2. In a large skillet, melt butter over medium heat. Add minced garlic and cook until fragrant.

3. Stir in flour and cook for 1-2 minutes until lightly golden, stirring constantly.

4. Gradually whisk in chicken broth and heavy cream until smooth and thickened.

5. Season with thyme, salt, and pepper.

6. Remove from heat and stir in shredded chicken, steamed broccoli, half of the cheddar cheese, and half of the mozzarella cheese.

7. Pour the mixture into the prepared baking dish. Sprinkle the remaining cheeses over the top.

8. Bake for 25-30 minutes, or until bubbly and golden on top.

9. Let it cool slightly before serving.

Nutritional Info (per serving):

Calories: 380

Protein: 30g

Carbohydrates: 8g

Fat: 25g

Fiber: 2g

Velvety Sweet Potato Puree

Servings: 4

Total Prep Time: 45 minutes

Ingredients:

- 2 large sweet potatoes, peeled and cubed
- 1/4 cup heavy cream
- 2 tbsp butter
- Salt and pepper to taste
- Optional: cinnamon or nutmeg for garnish

Directions:

1. Bring a large pot of water to a boil. Add the cubed sweet potatoes and cook until fork-tender, about 15-20 minutes.
2. Drain the sweet potatoes and return them to the pot.
3. Mash the sweet potatoes with a potato masher until smooth.

4. Stir in heavy cream and butter until well combined.

5. Season with salt and pepper to taste.

6. Serve hot, optionally garnished with a sprinkle of cinnamon or nutmeg.

Nutritional Info (per serving):

Calories: 220

Protein: 3g

Carbohydrates: 27g

Fat: 12g

Fiber: 4g

Smooth Cauliflower and Leek Mash

Servings: 4

Total Prep Time: 40 minutes

Ingredients:

- 1 large head cauliflower, cut into florets
- 2 leeks, white and light green parts only, chopped
- 2 cloves garlic, minced
- 1/4 cup heavy cream
- 2 tbsp butter
- Salt and pepper to taste

Directions:

1. Steam or boil cauliflower florets until very tender, about 10-15 minutes.
2. In a separate pan, melt butter over medium heat. Add chopped leeks and

minced garlic. Sauté until leeks are softened, about 5-7 minutes.

3. In a food processor or blender, combine the cooked cauliflower, sautéed leeks and garlic, heavy cream, and butter. Blend until smooth and creamy.

4. Season with salt and pepper to taste.

5. Serve hot as a side dish.

Nutritional Info (per serving):

Calories: 150

Protein: 4g

Carbohydrates: 12g

Fat: 10g

Fiber: 4g

Delicious Dinners

Creamy Chicken and Vegetable Puree

Servings: 4

Total Prep Time: 45 minutes

Ingredients:

- 1 lb boneless, skinless chicken breasts
- 2 cups mixed vegetables (carrots, peas, green beans)
- 1 onion, chopped
- 2 cloves garlic, minced
- 1 cup chicken broth
- 1/2 cup heavy cream
- Salt and pepper to taste

Directions:

1. Cook chicken breasts in a skillet until fully cooked. Remove and shred.

2. In the same skillet, sauté onions and garlic until softened.

3. Add mixed vegetables and cook until tender.

4. Pour in chicken broth and heavy cream. Simmer for 10-15 minutes.

5. Blend mixture until smooth using an immersion blender or transfer to a blender.

6. Season with salt and pepper to taste. Serve warm.

Nutritional Info:

(per serving)

Calories: 320

Fat: 18g

Carbohydrates: 12g

Protein: 25g

Savory Beef and Mushroom Puree

Servings: 4

Total Prep Time: 1 hour

Ingredients:

- 1 lb ground beef
- 8 oz mushrooms, sliced
- 1 onion, diced
- 2 cloves garlic, minced
- 1 cup beef broth
- 1/2 cup heavy cream
- Salt and pepper to taste

Directions:

1. Brown ground beef in a skillet until fully cooked. Drain excess fat.
2. Add onions and garlic, cook until softened.
3. Add mushrooms and cook until tender.

4. Pour in beef broth and heavy cream. Simmer for 15-20 minutes.

5. Blend mixture until smooth using an immersion blender or transfer to a blender.

6. Season with salt and pepper to taste. Serve warm.

Nutritional Info:

(per serving)

Calories: 380

Fat: 26g

Carbohydrates: 8g

Protein: 28g

Butternut Squash and Carrot Puree

Servings: 4

Total Prep Time: 40 minutes

Ingredients:

- 1 medium butternut squash, peeled, seeded, and cubed
- 2 large carrots, peeled and sliced
- 1 onion, chopped
- 2 cloves garlic, minced
- 4 cups vegetable broth
- 1/2 cup coconut milk
- Salt and pepper to taste

Directions:

1. Steam or boil butternut squash and carrots until very tender.

2. Sauté onions and garlic in a large pot until softened.

3. Add steamed squash and carrots to the pot along with vegetable broth.

4. Simmer for 10 minutes, then blend until smooth using an immersion blender or transfer to a blender.

5. Stir in coconut milk. Season with salt and pepper to taste. Serve warm.

Nutritional Info:

(per serving)

Calories: 220

Fat: 8g

Carbohydrates: 38g

Protein: 4g

Lentil and Spinach Puree

Servings: 4

Total Prep Time: 45 minutes

Ingredients:

- 1 cup dried green lentils, rinsed
- 1 onion, chopped
- 2 cloves garlic, minced
- 4 cups vegetable broth
- 2 cups fresh spinach
- 1/2 cup plain Greek yogurt
- Salt and pepper to taste

Directions:

1. Cook lentils in vegetable broth until tender, about 20-25 minutes.
2. Sauté onions and garlic until softened.
3. Add cooked lentils and spinach to the skillet. Cook until spinach wilts.

4. Blend mixture until smooth using an immersion blender or transfer to a blender.

5. Stir in Greek yogurt. Season with salt and pepper to taste. Serve warm.

Nutritional Info:

(per serving)

Calories: 280

Fat: 3g

Carbohydrates: 45g

Protein: 20g

Cheesy Chicken and Broccoli Bake

Servings: 6

Total Prep Time: 1 hour

Ingredients:

- 1 lb boneless, skinless chicken breasts, cooked and shredded
- 2 cups broccoli florets, steamed
- 1 onion, chopped
- 2 cloves garlic, minced
- 1 cup shredded cheddar cheese
- 1 cup milk
- 2 tbsp all-purpose flour
- Salt and pepper to taste

Directions:

1. Preheat oven to 375°F (190°C).
2. Sauté onions and garlic until softened.
3. In a bowl, whisk together milk and flour until smooth.

4. Add milk mixture to the skillet and cook until thickened.

5. Stir in shredded chicken, steamed broccoli, and half of the shredded cheese.

6. Transfer mixture to a baking dish. Top with remaining cheese.

7. Bake for 25-30 minutes or until bubbly and golden brown. Serve warm.

Nutritional Info:

(per serving)

Calories: 320

Fat: 15g

Carbohydrates: 14g

Protein: 30g

Soft Tuna Noodle Casserole

Servings: 4

Total Prep Time: 50 minutes

Ingredients:

- 8 oz egg noodles, cooked according to package instructions
- 2 cans (5 oz each) tuna, drained
- 1 cup frozen peas, thawed
- 1 onion, chopped
- 2 cloves garlic, minced
- 1 cup milk
- 1 cup shredded mozzarella cheese
- Salt and pepper to taste

Directions:

1. Preheat oven to 350°F (175°C).
2. Sauté onions and garlic until softened.
3. In a bowl, combine cooked egg noodles, tuna, peas, sautéed onions, garlic, milk,

and half of the shredded mozzarella cheese.

4. Transfer mixture to a baking dish. Top with remaining cheese.

5. Bake for 20-25 minutes or until heated through and cheese is melted. Serve warm.

Nutritional Info:

(per serving)

Calories: 380

Fat: 12g

Carbohydrates: 38g

Protein: 30g

Mild Beef and Vegetable Shepherd's Pie

Servings: 6

Total Prep Time: 1 hour 15 minutes

Ingredients:

- 1 lb ground beef
- 1 onion, chopped
- 2 cloves garlic, minced
- 2 cups mixed vegetables (corn, peas, carrots)
- 1 cup beef broth
- 2 cups mashed potatoes
- Salt and pepper to taste

Directions:

1. Preheat oven to 375°F (190°C).
2. Brown ground beef in a skillet until fully cooked. Drain excess fat.

3. Add onions and garlic, cook until softened.

4. Stir in mixed vegetables and beef broth. Simmer for 10 minutes.

5. Transfer beef mixture to a baking dish. Spread mashed potatoes evenly over the top.

6. Bake for 25-30 minutes or until potatoes are lightly browned. Serve warm.

Nutritional Info:

(per serving)

Calories: 380

Fat: 18g

Carbohydrates: 32g

Protein: 22g

Creamy Potato and Leek Bake

Servings: 4

Total Prep Time: 1 hour

Ingredients:

- 4 large potatoes, peeled and thinly sliced
- 2 leeks, white and light green parts only, sliced
- 1 cup heavy cream
- 1 cup shredded Gruyere cheese
- Salt and pepper to taste

Directions:

1. Preheat oven to 375°F (190°C).
2. Layer potato slices and leeks in a greased baking dish.
3. In a saucepan, heat heavy cream until just simmering. Pour over potatoes and leeks.

4. Sprinkle shredded Gruyere cheese over the top.

5. Bake for 45-50 minutes or until potatoes are tender and top is golden brown. Serve warm.

Nutritional Info:

(per serving)

Calories: 420

Fat: 28g

Carbohydrates: 30g

Protein: 12g

Smooth Salmon and Sweet Potato Puree

Servings: 4

Total Prep Time: 50 minutes

Ingredients:

- 1 lb salmon fillets
- 2 large sweet potatoes, peeled and cubed
- 1 onion, chopped
- 2 cloves garlic, minced
- 4 cups vegetable broth
- 1/2 cup coconut milk
- Salt and pepper to taste

Directions:

1. Bake or grill salmon until cooked through. Flake into small pieces.
2. Steam sweet potatoes until tender.
3. Sauté onions and garlic until softened.

4. Combine cooked sweet potatoes, onions, garlic, and vegetable broth in a pot. Simmer for 10 minutes.

5. Blend mixture until smooth using an immersion blender or transfer to a blender.

6. Stir in coconut milk and flaked salmon. Season with salt and pepper to taste. Serve warm.

Nutritional Info:

(per serving)

Calories: 340

Fat: 15g

Carbohydrates: 32g

Protein: 22g

Creamy Cod and Spinach Puree

Servings: 4

Total Prep Time: 30 minutes

Ingredients:

- 4 cod fillets, skinless and boneless
- 1 lb fresh spinach, washed and trimmed
- 1 onion, finely chopped
- 2 cloves garlic, minced
- 1 cup heavy cream
- 1/2 cup chicken or vegetable broth
- 2 tablespoons olive oil
- Salt and pepper to taste
- Fresh parsley for garnish (optional)

Directions:

1. In a large skillet, heat olive oil over medium heat. Add chopped onion and garlic, and sauté until softened, about 3-4 minutes.

2. Add spinach to the skillet in batches, stirring until wilted. Cook until spinach is completely wilted and excess moisture has evaporated, about 5-7 minutes. Remove from heat and set aside.

3. In another skillet, heat a little olive oil over medium-high heat. Season cod fillets with salt and pepper, then add them to the skillet. Cook for 3-4 minutes per side, until fish is opaque and flakes easily with a fork. Remove from heat and set aside.

4. In a blender or food processor, combine the cooked spinach mixture, heavy cream, and chicken or vegetable broth. Blend until smooth and creamy.

5. Transfer the spinach puree back to the skillet. Heat over medium heat until warmed through, stirring occasionally.

6. Serve the cod fillets over the creamy spinach puree. Garnish with fresh parsley if desired.

Nutritional Info (per serving):

Calories: 380 kcal

Protein: 28g

Fat: 25g

Carbohydrates: 11g

Fiber: 4g

Sugar: 3g

Sodium: 310mg

Snacks and Small Bites

Soft Avocado and Banana Bites

Servings: Makes about 12 bites

Total Prep Time: 15 minutes

Ingredients:

- 1 ripe avocado
- 1 ripe banana
- 1 tablespoon honey (optional)

Directions:

1. Mash the avocado and banana together until smooth.
2. Stir in honey if desired.
3. Spoon mixture into bite-sized molds or onto parchment paper.
4. Freeze for 1-2 hours until firm.

Nutritional Info: (Per bite) Calories: 35, Fat: 2g, Carbohydrates: 5g, Protein: 0.5g

Mini Quinoa Patties

Servings: Makes about 12 patties

Total Prep Time: 30 minutes

Ingredients:

- 1 cup cooked quinoa
- 1/2 cup grated cheese (such as cheddar)
- 1/4 cup breadcrumbs
- 1 egg, beaten
- Salt and pepper to taste

Directions:

1. Preheat oven to 375°F (190°C) and line a baking sheet with parchment paper.
2. In a bowl, mix together all ingredients until well combined.
3. Form mixture into small patties and place on the baking sheet.
4. Bake for 15-20 minutes until golden brown and crispy.

Nutritional Info: (Per patty) Calories: 60, Fat: 3g, Carbohydrates: 6g, Protein: 3g

Sweet Potato and Carrot Fritters

Servings: Makes about 10 fritters

Total Prep Time: 40 minutes

Ingredients:

- 1 medium sweet potato, grated
- 1 large carrot, grated
- 1/4 cup flour (can use gluten-free flour)
- 1 egg, beaten
- 1/2 teaspoon ground cumin
- Salt and pepper to taste

Directions:

1. In a bowl, mix together grated sweet potato, carrot, flour, egg, cumin, salt, and pepper.
2. Heat oil in a skillet over medium heat.
3. Spoon mixture into the skillet, flattening with a spatula to form fritters.

4. Cook for 3-4 minutes on each side until golden brown and cooked through.

Nutritional Info: (Per fritter) Calories: 50, Fat: 1g, Carbohydrates: 9g, Protein: 2g

Creamy Spinach and Artichoke Dip

Servings: Serves 6-8

Total Prep Time: 25 minutes

Ingredients:

- 1 (10 oz) package frozen spinach, thawed and drained
- 1 (14 oz) can artichoke hearts, drained and chopped
- 1 cup grated Parmesan cheese
- 1 cup sour cream
- 1/2 cup mayonnaise
- 1 clove garlic, minced

Directions:

1. Preheat oven to 350°F (175°C).
2. In a mixing bowl, combine all ingredients until well mixed.

3. Transfer mixture to a baking dish.

4. Bake for 20 minutes until bubbly and golden on top.

Nutritional Info: (Per serving) Calories: 180, Fat: 15g, Carbohydrates: 6g, Protein: 6g

Silky Hummus

Servings: Makes about 2 cups

Total Prep Time: 10 minutes

Ingredients:

- 1 (15 oz) can chickpeas, drained and rinsed
- 1/4 cup tahini
- 2 tablespoons lemon juice
- 1 clove garlic, minced
- 1/4 teaspoon ground cumin
- Salt and pepper to taste

Directions:

1. In a food processor, blend all ingredients until smooth.
2. If too thick, add water, 1 tablespoon at a time, until desired consistency is reached.
3. Adjust seasoning to taste.

Nutritional Info: (Per 2 tablespoon serving) Calories: 50, Fat: 3g, Carbohydrates: 5g, Protein: 2g

Smooth Avocado Yogurt Dip

Servings: Makes about 1 cup

Total Prep Time: 10 minutes

Ingredients:

- 1 ripe avocado
- 1/2 cup plain Greek yogurt
- 1 tablespoon lime juice
- 1 clove garlic, minced
- Salt and pepper to taste

Directions:

1. In a blender or food processor, combine all ingredients until smooth.
2. Adjust seasoning to taste.
3. Serve chilled with vegetables or chips.

Nutritional Info: (Per 2 tablespoon serving) Calories: 30, Fat: 2g, Carbohydrates: 2g, Protein: 1g

Soft Cinnamon Applesauce Bites

Servings: Makes about 24 bites

Total Prep Time: 20 minutes

Ingredients:

- 2 cups unsweetened applesauce
- 1 tablespoon cinnamon
- 1 tablespoon honey (optional)

Directions:

1. In a bowl, mix together applesauce, cinnamon, and honey (if using).
2. Spoon mixture into silicone candy molds or ice cube trays.
3. Freeze for 2 hours until firm.

Nutritional Info: (Per bite) Calories: 15, Fat: 0g, Carbohydrates: 4g, Protein: 0g

Creamy Banana Pudding

Servings: Serves 4-6

Total Prep Time: 20 minutes

Ingredients:

- 2 ripe bananas, mashed
- 1 cup milk (dairy or plant-based)
- 2 tablespoons cornstarch
- 2 tablespoons honey or maple syrup
- 1 teaspoon vanilla extract

Directions:

1. In a saucepan, whisk together milk and cornstarch over medium heat until thickened.
2. Remove from heat and stir in mashed bananas, honey (or maple syrup), and vanilla extract.
3. Pour into serving dishes and refrigerate until chilled.

Nutritional Info: (Per serving) Calories: 120,
Fat: 1g, Carbohydrates: 27g, Protein: 2g

Peanut Butter Mousse

Servings: Serves 4

Total Prep Time: 15 minutes + chilling time

Ingredients:

- 1 cup creamy peanut butter
- 1/4 cup honey or maple syrup
- 1 teaspoon vanilla extract
- 1 cup heavy cream, whipped

Directions:

1. In a bowl, mix together peanut butter, honey (or maple syrup), and vanilla extract until smooth.
2. Gently fold in whipped cream until well combined.
3. Divide into serving dishes and chill for at least 2 hours.

Nutritional Info: (Per serving) Calories: 480, Fat: 39g, Carbohydrates: 22g, Protein: 14g

Soft Blueberry Muffins

Servings: Makes 12 muffins

Total Prep Time: 30 minutes

Ingredients:

- 2 cups all-purpose flour
- 1/2 cup sugar
- 1 tablespoon baking powder
- 1/2 teaspoon salt
- 1/2 cup unsalted butter, melted
- 1 cup milk
- 2 eggs
- 1 teaspoon vanilla extract
- 1 cup fresh or frozen blueberries

Directions:

1. Preheat oven to 375°F (190°C) and line a muffin tin with paper liners.
2. In a large bowl, whisk together flour, sugar, baking powder, and salt.

3. In another bowl, whisk together melted butter, milk, eggs, and vanilla extract.

4. Pour wet ingredients into dry ingredients and stir until just combined.

5. Gently fold in blueberries.

6. Divide batter evenly among muffin cups.

7. Bake for 20-25 minutes until golden brown and a toothpick inserted into the center comes out clean.

Nutritional Info: (Per muffin) Calories: 200, Fat: 8g, Carbohydrates: 28g, Protein: 4g

Hydration and Desserts

Creamy Banana and Avocado Smoothie

Servings: 2

Total Prep Time: 5 minutes

Ingredients:

- 1 ripe banana, peeled and sliced
- 1/2 ripe avocado, peeled and pitted
- 1 cup milk (dairy or plant-based)
- 1 tablespoon honey or maple syrup (optional)
- 1/2 teaspoon vanilla extract
- Ice cubes (optional)

Directions:

1. Place all ingredients in a blender.
2. Blend until smooth and creamy.
3. Taste and adjust sweetness if necessary.

4. Pour into glasses and serve immediately.

Nutritional Info: (per serving)

Calories: 200

Protein: 4g

Fat: 9g

Carbohydrates: 28g

Fiber: 5g

Blueberry Greek Yogurt Smoothie

Servings: 2

Total Prep Time: 7 minutes

Ingredients:

- 1 cup fresh or frozen blueberries
- 1 cup Greek yogurt
- 1/2 cup milk (dairy or plant-based)
- 1 tablespoon honey or maple syrup (optional)
- 1/2 teaspoon vanilla extract

Directions:

1. Combine all ingredients in a blender.
2. Blend until smooth and creamy.
3. Adjust sweetness if desired.
4. Pour into glasses and serve immediately.

Nutritional Info: (per serving)

Calories: 180

Protein: 12g

Fat: 3g

Carbohydrates: 28g

Fiber: 3g

Peach and Almond Milk Smoothie

Servings: 2

Total Prep Time: 5 minutes

Ingredients:

- 2 ripe peaches, peeled and sliced
- 1 cup almond milk (or any milk of choice)
- 1/2 cup plain Greek yogurt
- 1 tablespoon honey or maple syrup (optional)
- 1/2 teaspoon almond extract (optional)

Directions:

1. Place all ingredients in a blender.
2. Blend until smooth and creamy.
3. Taste and adjust sweetness or almond flavoring.
4. Pour into glasses and serve immediately.

Nutritional Info: (per serving)

Calories: 160

Protein: 8g

Fat: 3g

Carbohydrates: 30g

Fiber: 3g

Protein-Packed Peanut Butter and Chocolate Shake

Servings: 1

Total Prep Time: 5 minutes

Ingredients:

- 1 ripe banana
- 1 cup milk (dairy or plant-based)
- 1 scoop chocolate protein powder
- 2 tablespoons natural peanut butter
- Ice cubes (optional)

Directions:

1. Combine all ingredients in a blender.
2. Blend until smooth and creamy.
3. Add ice cubes if desired for a colder shake.
4. Pour into a glass and serve immediately.

Nutritional Info: (per serving)

Calories: 450

Protein: 30g

Fat: 18g

Carbohydrates: 45g

Fiber: 6g

Soft Baked Apple Cinnamon Crumble

Servings: 6

Total Prep Time: 40 minutes

Ingredients:

- 4 large apples, peeled, cored, and sliced
- 1 tablespoon lemon juice
- 1/2 cup rolled oats
- 1/4 cup all-purpose flour
- 1/4 cup brown sugar
- 1/2 teaspoon ground cinnamon
- 1/4 cup butter, melted

Directions:

1. Preheat oven to 350°F (175°C). Grease a baking dish.
2. Toss apple slices with lemon juice and spread evenly in the baking dish.

3. In a bowl, combine oats, flour, brown sugar, cinnamon, and melted butter until crumbly.

4. Sprinkle the oat mixture over the apples.

5. Bake for 30 minutes or until the topping is golden brown and apples are tender.

6. Serve warm with a scoop of vanilla ice cream if desired.

Nutritional Info: (per serving)

Calories: 250

Protein: 2g

Fat: 9g

Carbohydrates: 42g

Fiber: 5g

Creamy Cheesecake Cups

Servings: 12

Total Prep Time: 30 minutes + chilling time

Ingredients:

- 12 graham cracker squares
- 16 oz cream cheese, softened
- 1/2 cup granulated sugar
- 1 teaspoon vanilla extract
- 2 large eggs
- Fresh berries or fruit compote for topping (optional)

Directions:

1. Preheat oven to 325°F (165°C). Line a muffin tin with paper liners.
2. Place a graham cracker square in each muffin cup.
3. In a mixing bowl, beat cream cheese, sugar, and vanilla until smooth.

4. Add eggs one at a time, mixing well after each addition.

5. Spoon cream cheese mixture over graham cracker bases.

6. Bake for 20 minutes or until centers are almost set.

7. Cool completely at room temperature, then refrigerate for at least 2 hours.

8. Top with fresh berries or fruit compote before serving, if desired.

Nutritional Info: (per serving)

Calories: 250

Protein: 5g

Fat: 18g

Carbohydrates: 18g

Fiber: 0.5g

Vanilla Bean Pudding

Servings: 4

Total Prep Time: 20 minutes + chilling time

Ingredients:

- 2 cups whole milk
- 1/2 cup granulated sugar
- 3 tablespoons cornstarch
- 1/4 teaspoon salt
- 1 vanilla bean, split and scraped (or 1 teaspoon vanilla extract)

Directions:

1. In a saucepan, whisk together milk, sugar, cornstarch, and salt.
2. Add vanilla bean seeds and pod (or vanilla extract).
3. Heat over medium heat, stirring constantly until mixture thickens and boils.

4. Boil for 1 minute, then remove from heat.

5. Remove vanilla bean pod if used.

6. Pour into serving dishes.

7. Cover with plastic wrap directly on the surface of the pudding to prevent a skin from forming.

8. Chill in the refrigerator until set, about 2 hours.

Nutritional Info: (per serving)

Calories: 250

Protein: 5g

Fat: 7g

Carbohydrates: 41g

Fiber: 0g

Fruit-Infused Gelatin

Servings: 6

Total Prep Time: 4 hours (including chilling time)

Ingredients:

- 1 package (3 oz) flavored gelatin (choose your favorite fruit flavor)
- 2 cups boiling water
- 1 cup cold water
- Fresh fruit slices (optional)

Directions:

1. In a bowl, dissolve gelatin in boiling water.
2. Stir in cold water.
3. Pour into a mold or individual serving dishes.
4. Chill in the refrigerator until set, about 4 hours or overnight.

5. Serve with fresh fruit slices if desired.

Nutritional Info: (per serving)

Calories: 80

Protein: 2g

Fat: 0g

Carbohydrates: 18g

Fiber: 0g

Chocolate Avocado Pudding

Servings: 4

Total Prep Time: 10 minutes + chilling time

Ingredients:

- 2 ripe avocados, peeled and pitted
- 1/2 cup cocoa powder
- 1/2 cup honey or maple syrup
- 1/3 cup milk (dairy or plant-based)
- 1 teaspoon vanilla extract

Directions:

1. In a food processor or blender, combine all ingredients.
2. Blend until smooth and creamy.
3. Taste and adjust sweetness if desired.
4. Divide into serving dishes.
5. Chill in the refrigerator for at least 2 hours before serving.

Nutritional Info: (per serving)

Calories: 300

Protein: 4g

Fat: 15g

Carbohydrates: 45g

Fiber: 10g

Moist Carrot Cake with Cream Cheese Frosting

Servings: 12 slices

Total Prep Time: 1 hour 30 minutes

Ingredients:

For the Carrot Cake:

- 2 cups all-purpose flour
- 2 cups granulated sugar
- 1 teaspoon baking powder
- 1 teaspoon baking soda
- 1 teaspoon salt
- 1 teaspoon ground cinnamon
- 4 large eggs
- 1 cup vegetable oil
- 1 teaspoon vanilla extract
- 3 cups grated carrots (about 4-5 medium carrots)

- 1 cup chopped walnuts or pecans (optional)
- For the Cream Cheese Frosting:
- 8 ounces cream cheese, softened
- 1/2 cup unsalted butter, softened
- 4 cups powdered sugar
- 1 teaspoon vanilla extract

Directions:

1. Preheat your oven to 350°F (175°C). Grease and flour two 9-inch round cake pans, or line them with parchment paper.
2. In a large bowl, whisk together the flour, sugar, baking powder, baking soda, salt, and cinnamon until well combined.
3. In another bowl, beat the eggs, vegetable oil, and vanilla extract until smooth.
4. Gradually add the wet ingredients to the dry ingredients, mixing until just combined.

5. Fold in the grated carrots and chopped nuts (if using) until evenly distributed in the batter.

6. Divide the batter evenly between the prepared cake pans.

7. Bake in the preheated oven for 30-35 minutes, or until a toothpick inserted into the center comes out clean.

8. Remove from the oven and allow the cakes to cool in the pans for 10 minutes before transferring them to a wire rack to cool completely.

9. In a large bowl, beat together the softened cream cheese and butter until smooth and creamy.

10. Gradually add the powdered sugar, one cup at a time, beating well after each addition.

11. Stir in the vanilla extract and beat the frosting until light and fluffy.

12. Once the cakes are completely cool, place one cake layer on a serving plate or cake stand.

13. Spread a layer of cream cheese frosting over the top.

14. Place the second cake layer on top and frost the top and sides of the cake with the remaining frosting.

15. Slice and serve the carrot cake immediately, or store it in the refrigerator until ready to serve.

Nutritional Information (per serving):

Calories: 560 kcal

Total Fat: 30g

Saturated Fat: 10g

Trans Fat: 0g

Cholesterol: 100mg

Sodium: 380mg

Total Carbohydrate: 70g

Dietary Fiber: 2g

Sugars: 52g

Protein: 6g